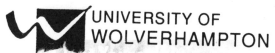

UNIVERSITY OF WOLVERHAMPTON

Clinical
Pharmacology

for Nurses

D0618829

For Churchill Livingstone

Commissioning editor: Ellen Green
Project manager: Valerie Burgess
Project controller: Pat Miller
Design direction: Judith Wright
Copy editor: Anne Horscroft
Sales promotion executive: Hilary Brown

Test Yourself in

Clinical
Pharmacology
for Nurses

John Trounce MD FRCP
Professor Emeritus of Clinical Pharmacology, Guy's Hospital
Medical School; Physician Emeritus, Guy's Hospital, London, UK

Dinah Gould BSc, MPhil, PhD, DipN, RGN, RNT
Senior Lecturer in Nursing Studies, King's College, London, UK

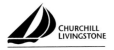
CHURCHILL
LIVINGSTONE

NEW YORK EDINBURGH LONDON MADRID MELBOURNE SAN FRANCISCO TOKYO 1997

CHURCHILL LIVINGSTONE
Medical Division of Pearson Professional Limited

Distributed in the United States of America by Churchill Livingstone, 650 Avenue of the Americas, New York, N.Y. 10011, and by associated companies, branches and representatives throughout the world.

First published 1997

ISBN 0 443 05783 4

British Library Cataloguing in Publication Data
A catalogue record for this book is available from the British Library.

Library of Congress Cataloging in Publication Data
A catalog record for this book is available from the Library of Congress.

Note
Medical knowledge is constantly changing. As new information becomes available, changes in treatment, procedures, equipment and the use of drugs become necessary. The editors/authors/contributors and the publishers have, as far as it is possible, taken care to ensure that the information given in this text is accurate and up-to-date. However, readers are strongly advised to confirm that the information, especially with regard to drug usage, complies with latest legislation and standards of practice.

Printed by Bell and Bain Ltd., Glasgow

Contents

Acknowledgements

We thank Dr M. B. Barnett, Lynette Stone and
Mr D. M. Watson for their help and advice.

Note

During 1997 the British Approved Nomenclature (BAN) for drugs will be replaced by the rINN system and will involve name changes for some drugs. In this text the rINN name is given in parentheses after the British Approved Name where an alteration has occurred.

Introduction

Multiple choice questions (MCQs) are an effective method of revising and consolidating knowledge. Clinical pharmacology is an ideal subject to test in this way because the information required is precise. With the increasing trend towards nurse prescribing and nurses' expanding role in the administration of complex treatment regimens and monitoring the outcome of drug treatment, it is important they should be confident with all aspects of drug action and use.

The questions in this book have been designed to provide a combination of practical, everyday problems and to explore some of the more theoretical aspects of clinical pharmacology. Both are based on *Clinical Pharmacology for Nurses* (15th edition) published by Churchill Livingstone. However, sufficient detail is given on the answer pages for this book to be used alone. The questions are divided into sections, each preceded by an introductory paragraph. We have adopted the traditional format used with MCQs. The stem question is followed by five possible answers, of which any number may be true or false. The correct answers are given on the following page. For those who wish to award themselves marks to assess progress, a common system is:

A true answer = score +2
A false answer = score −1
No answer = score 0

A typical pass mark in an examination composed entirely of MCQs is 50%. An arbitrary pass mark fails to take into account the seniority of the nurse and the amount of clinical pharmacology included in the teaching programme, so it may require modification. It must be stressed, however, that the main purpose of this book is educational. The series of questions, designed by a professor of clinical pharmacology and a senior nurse educationalist, is intended to stimulate nurses' interest in drugs and to facilitate the learning process. It should also provide a useful method of updating for qualified nurses who feel the need to revise their knowledge of clinical pharmacology. The questions may be tackled by working through the book in order or by picking individual sections to test knowledge in specific areas.

The book will also be a valuable resource for lecturers. Setting and marking examinations using MCQs allows the exploration of a wide range of knowledge, while marking is rapid and free from subjective bias.

We have made every effort to ensure that the information in this book is correct at the time of publication. Drug schedules and usage are constantly changing and important adverse effects emerge. Readers may disagree with some of our recommendations because in some areas of medical and nursing practice there are no absolute rules. We hope that this will stimulate discussion and research. However, errors may have occurred. When in doubt, the manufacturer's data sheet or some other authoritative source should be consulted.

General principles

Pharmacology is concerned with the mode of action of drugs. Clinical pharmacology deals with drug action in humans and particularly, in the treatment of disease. It covers not only the therapeutic action of drugs, but also their absorption, distribution throughout the body and their elimination.

If a drug is to be of maximum benefit to the patient, the method of administration and mode of action must be taken into consideration. Therefore a grasp of the principles of clinical pharmacology is essential before the use of individual groups of drugs can be fully appreciated. The nurse responsible for drug administration needs to be conversant with dosage schedules, duration of action and the appropriate routes of administration. The questions in this section are concerned with the absorption and metabolism of drugs, factors influencing the dosage regimen and factors which can modify the patient's response to drugs.

1

When a drug is said to have low bioavailability if given by mouth, this means:

a. Only a small proportion of the dose enters the circulation
b. It may be broken down extensively as it passes from the gut and through the liver
c. It may be effective if chewed rather than swallowed
d. It should be given as slow-release capsules
e. It is likely to be ineffective if given by mouth

2

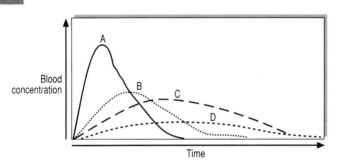

The concentration of a drug in the bloodstream is a good indication of whether the correct dose is being given to produce the required therapeutic effect. The graph above illustrates the plasma concentration of a drug administered by different routes, plotted against time. Circle the appropriate letter:

a. By mouth – A B C D
b. Intravenous – A B C D
c. Intramuscular – A B C D
d. By mouth with large first-pass effect – A B C D
e. Intramuscular with first-pass effect – A B C D

1

a. **True**
b. **True**
c. **True** – If chewed, the drug is absorbed from the mouth and bypasses the liver
d. **False** – It would be broken down before it reached the circulation
e. **True**

2

a. **By mouth** – C
b. **Intravenous** – A
c. **Intramuscular** – B
d. **By mouth with first-pass effect** – D
e. **Intramuscular with first-pass effect** – B

3

After absorption into the circulation, drugs may be significantly eliminated:

a. Via the lungs
b. By being broken down in the liver
c. By being excreted by the kidneys
d. Via the skin
e. Into the bowel

4

A drug has a half-life of 6 hours. This represents:

a. Half the time it is effective
b. The time taken for the blood level to halve after a single dose
c. Half the time it may be kept in storage
d. Half the lethal dose
e. The time it takes to be completely eliminated

5

Drugs with a long half-life:

a. Require frequent dosing to keep the blood levels steady
b. Require repeated dosing over several days to reach a steady blood concentration
c. Are eliminated slowly
d. Can only be given by mouth
e. Are likely to be less effective therapeutically

6

Several factors influence the dosage of a drug. For example, a patient has been prescribed injections of morphine to relieve pain. The size of the doses will be determined by:

a. The ethnic origin of the patient
b. Genetic factors
c. The patient's liver function
d. The severity of the pain
e. The patient's renal function

3

a. **True**
b. **True**
c. **True**
d. **False** – Although drugs can penetrate the skin
e. **True** – Rarely via the bile or into the bowel

4

a. **False**
b. **True**
c. **False**
d. **False**
e. **False** – Half-life also gives a rough idea of how long a drug is effective and, therefore, the frequency of dosage required

5

a. **False** – Require *less* rather than *more* frequent dosage
b. **True** – They require administration over five half-lives to reach a steady state
c. **True**
d. **False**
e. **False**

6

a. **False**
b. **False** – But may be true for some drugs
c. **True** – Morphine is broken down by the liver and accumulation can occur in patients with liver disease
d. **True**
e. **True** – An active breakdown product of morphine is excreted by the kidney and in patients with renal failure accumulation can occur

7

Some drugs should be given before meals:

a. To decrease the first-pass effect
b. To aid absorption
c. To prevent diarrhoea
d. To obtain a high concentration of the drug in the intestine
e. To avoid gastric irritation

8

The following drugs are taken with or after food:

a. Erythromycin
b. Non-steroidal anti-inflammatory agents (NSAIAs)
c. Corticosteroids
d. Sodium valproate
e. Tetracycline

9

Certain drugs are absorbed into the circulation through the skin and may be used in this way. These include:

a. Estrogens
b. Hyoscine
c. Salbutamol
d. Glyceryl trinitrate
e. Some NSAIAs

7

a. **False**
b. **True**
c. **False**
d. **True** – Certain anthelmintics (e.g. niclosamide) are given in this way
e. **False** – Irritant drugs are often given with or after food

8

a. **True** – Reduces indigestion and nausea
b. **True** – Reduces gastric irritation
c. **True** – Best with food or milk to reduce adverse gastrointestinal symptoms
d. **True** – Reduces indigestion
e. **False** – Certain foods may reduce absorption

In general, absorption is better with many drugs when taken fasting. Irritant drugs usually given with or after food

9

a. **True** – Given in this way for hormone replacement treatment
b. **True** – In the prevention of motion sickness
c. **False**
d. **True** – Used in patients with angina, but dose control is difficult
e. **True** – Applied as ointment over joints, but efficacy is doubtful

10

Drugs often act on receptors in tissues. If they activate the receptor they are termed agonists; if they block the receptor, preventing activation, they are termed antagonists. Which of the following are true?

a. Salbutamol is an agonist
b. Morphine is an antagonist
c. Dopamine is an agonist
d. Propranolol is an antagonist
e. Aluminium hydroxide is an antagonist

11

Enzymes are naturally occurring substances which increase the rate of chemical reactions. Enzyme inhibition by drugs plays an important part in some aspects of therapeutics. Which?

a. Elimination of drugs by the liver
b. Penetration of drugs into cells
c. Modifying the function of certain cells
d. Destruction of some types of malignant cells
e. Destruction of bacteria

12

To obtain maximum efficacy and to avoid toxic effects, the dose of a few drugs is partly controlled by repeated measurements of the blood concentration. Which of the following drugs require this kind of monitoring?

a. Amoxycillin
b. Gentamicin
c. Morphine
d. Lithium
e. Phenytoin

10

a. **True** – A β_2 receptor agonist which dilates the bronchi
b. **False** – Activates receptors in the nervous system which suppress pain
c. **True** – Levodopa is converted to dopamine, which stimulates receptors in the brain and relieves Parkinson's disease
d. **True** – Blocks β receptors in the sympathetic system, slows the heart rate and reduces blood pressure
e. **False** – No effect on receptors

11

a. **True**
b. **False**
c. **True**
d. **True** – By inhibiting enzymes in malignant cells or bacteria
e. **True** – By inhibiting enzymes in malignant cells or bacteria

12

a. **False**
b. **True** – Levels before and after dosing
c. **False**
d. **True**
e. **True**

13

An oral syringe to measure liquid drugs:

a. Can contain up to 10 ml
b. Can contain up to 5.0 ml
c. Is marked in 1.0 ml divisions
d. Is marked in 0.5 ml divisions
e. Should be used for doses of 5.0–10 ml

14

What is the maximum volume that should be given as a single intramuscular injection at one site?

a. 1.0 ml
b. 2.0 ml
c. 5.0 ml
d. 10 ml
e. 20 ml

15

Using a standard intravenous giving set, the volume of 20 macrodrops of crystalloid is?

a. 0.25 ml
b. 0.5 ml
c. 1.0 ml
d. 2.0 ml
e. 5.0 ml

13

a. **False**
b. **True**
c. **False**
d. **True**
e. **False** – Should be used for doses up to 5.0 ml: a 5.0 ml spoon is used for larger doses

14

a. **False**
b. **False**
c. **True**
d. **False** – Can cause pain
e. **False** – Can cause pain

15

a. **False**
b. **False**
c. **True**
d. **False**
e. **False**

The role of nurses in drug administration

Drug therapy plays a major part in the treatment of patients in hospital and in the community. In most instances drugs are prescribed by a doctor and dispensed by a pharmacist, but it is the responsibility of nurses to ensure safe and reliable administration, monitor side-effects and to secure the co-operation of patients in taking their drugs. This section explores each of these issues, with emphasis on the need for safety at all times.

Patient management is now recognized as a team activity and this team may well include a pharmacist whose close co-operation with the nursing staff can be of great mutual benefit.

In the future, nurses will have an increasing role in prescribing. This may require some modification of the present regulations governing the use of drugs.

16

A 65-year-old carpenter has been admitted to your ward for minor surgery. You are responsible for his post-operative care. He says that he is in pain and feels nauseated. According to his prescription sheet he can be given both an analgesic and an anti-emetic drug, but the house doctor has not signed the prescription for the painkiller. Which of the following would be the correct action?

a. Give both injections because the patient is suffering pain and nausea
b. Give only the anti-emetic drug as the house doctor has not signed for the analgesic
c. Contact the house doctor so that the analgesic is properly prescribed, then give both drugs
d. Give both injections, then contact the house doctor so the analgesic may be properly prescribed
e. Give the injections and speak to the consultant later

17

Having resolved the difficulties associated with your patient's prescription, you prepare the injections. The analgesic is a controlled drug. The correct procedure for administration must include:

a. Two people checking the drug
b. Two people checking the drug, with both present when it is administered
c. Two people checking the drug, with both present when it is administered and both signing the controlled drug book at the patient's bedside in his presence
d. Two people signing the controlled drug book at the bedside, in the patient's presence
e. The injection must be checked by the ward sister

16

a. **False**
b. **False**
c. **True**
d. **False**
e. **False**

17

a. **False**
b. **False**
c. **True**
d. **False**
e. **False**

18

Which sites can be used to administer intramuscular injections?

a. The outer aspect of the upper arm, middle third space between the knee and greater trochanter and the upper, outer quadrant of the buttock
b. The upper, outer quadrant of the buttock only
c. The abdominal wall
d. The calf muscle
e. None of the above

19

When your patient has recovered sufficiently to drink clear fluids, you decide that he should be able to take his usual drugs by mouth. He refuses to swallow the tablets, saying they will make him feel sick again. Which is the correct action to take?

a. Leave the tablets with him so he can take them later
b. Dispose of the tablets down the lavatory
c. Mark the drug chart to the effect that they have not been taken
d. Dispose of the tablets down the lavatory and mark the drug chart to show that they have not been taken
e. None of the above

20

A frail, elderly man who lives alone is admitted after falling and fracturing his femur. He is anxious and confused, thinking he is alone in a wood and has seen a fairy. You are asked to prepare him for theatre. This involves giving him a subcutaneous injection. Which sites are usually used to administer a drug subcutaneously?

a. The outer aspect of the upper arm
b. The outer aspect of the thigh
c. The dorsum of the hand
d. The skin of the abdominal wall
e. The chest wall

18

a. **True**
b. **False**
c. **False** – Used only for certain subcutaneous injections
d. **False**
e. **False**

19

a. **False**
b. **False**
c. **False**
d. **True**
e. **False**

20

a. **True**
b. **True**
c. **False**
d. **True**
e. **False**

21

Which categories of drugs are frequently administered by the intravenous route?

a. Heparin
b. Thrombolytic drugs
c. Cytotoxic drugs
d. Anthelmintic drugs
e. Warfarin

22

A patient's sister arrives on the ward with a bottle containing his usual drugs. The bottle contains three different types of tablet and is unlabelled. Neither the patient nor his sister can explain what the tablets are for. What is the fate of these drugs?

a. To be destroyed
b. To be placed on the drug trolley to be dispensed at the next round
c. To be stored in the ward medicine cupboard until he goes home
d. To be given to his sister so she can keep them safely until he goes home
e. To be sent to the pharmacy for identification

23

Which of the following are correct?

a. Unused drugs may be returned from the ward to the pharmacy for checking and use
b. Drugs given by mouth should be swallowed, if possible, with the patient sitting up
c. Drugs which are eliminated rapidly (short half-life) are least likely to have their therapeutic effect impaired by poor compliance
d. Nurses have a responsibility to teach patients about their drugs before they are discharged
e. Nurses working in the community may hold a stock of controlled drugs

21

a. **True**
b. **True**
c. **True**
d. **False** – By mouth
e. **False** – By mouth

22

a. **True**
b. **False**
c. **False**
d. **False**
e. **False**

23

a. **True**
b. **True**
c. **False** – Slowly eliminated drugs are preferable if compliance is poor
d. **True**
e. **False** – A stock of controlled drugs can only be held in hospital

24

The hospital pharmacy can:

a. Supply drugs for use on the ward
b. Advise on the storage of drugs
c. Advise on the preparation of drugs
d. Prescribe drugs
e. Provide information on the side-effects of drugs

25

The British National Formulary:

a. Lists only those drugs thought to be 'best buys'
b. Gives no guidance on treatment
c. Lists important interactions between drugs
d. Includes the Nurse Prescriber Formulary
e. Is published annually

24

a. **True**
b. **True**
c. **True**
d. **False**
e. **True**

25

a. **False** – Lists approved and proprietary drugs available in the UK
b. **False** – Restricted, but useful, guidance on treatment is included
c. **True**
d. **True**
e. **False** – Published twice a year

The autonomic nervous system, asthma and migraine

The autonomic nervous system (ANS) is responsible for controlling involuntary actions – those which occur without our conscious effort and of which, under normal circumstances, we are unaware. The ANS controls the action of the gastrointestinal (GI) tract and respiration. It also helps to control blood pressure through its action on the muscular layer in the walls of the arteries. The activity of the ANS can be modified by many drugs, so it is necessary to understand its functions.

One of the most important uses of drugs which modify the actions of the ANS is in the treatment of **asthma**. Nurses play an important part in the care of patients with asthma, and as the incidence of this disorder is growing, it is likely that this group will represent an increasing part of the caseload of nurses in the future. Patients, many of whom are young, need help to cope with a chronic disease which may be potentially life-threatening. Nurses must monitor symptoms, identify triggering factors and teach the patient and family how and when to administer the required drugs.

Drugs affecting the ANS are used in other conditions including hypertension, for premedication, and in disorders of motility of the GI tract. They are considered in the relevant sections.

Although **migraine** attacks are not life-threatening, they are very debilitating. A range of drugs can be used to control migraine, and when taken properly, allow most sufferers to lead a normal life.

26

You and a junior colleague are to look after an extremely nervous patient. In preparation, you ensure that your colleague fully appreciates the function of the autonomic nervous system because, not only is it concerned with most visceral activities, but it plays a large part in the response to stress and anxiety. Which of the following are true?

a. The autonomic system supplies the gastrointestinal tract, the respiratory system, the urogenital organs and all voluntary muscles
b. The autonomic nervous system has sensory as well as motor functions
c. The autonomic system consists of two divisions, usually having opposite actions
d. The sympathetic system consists of chains of ganglia lying on one side of the spinal cord only
e. The ganglia of the parasympathetic nervous system are situated near the organs which they supply

27

Which of the following statements are true?

a. Transmission of impulses between adjacent nerves is a chemical event
b. The above is due to the release of a chemical transmitter at the nerve ending
c. When the parasympathetic nervous system is stimulated acetylcholine is liberated
d. When the sympathetic nervous system is stimulated cholinesterase is liberated
e. Acetylcholine acts as a transmitter in the brain as well as in the autonomic nervous system

26

a. **False** – The autonomic nervous system supplies the gastrointestinal tract, respiratory system and urogenital organs, but not the voluntary muscles

b. **True** – The autonomic nervous system may form reflexes in the spinal cord or sensation may reach higher centres

c. **True** – The autonomic nervous system consists of the parasympathetic and sympathetic systems

d. **False** – The sympathetic system consists of chains of ganglia lying on both sides of the vertebral column and connected to the spinal cord

e. **True** – The nerve fibres are distributed with cranial nerves III, VII, IX and X and with the sacral nerve

27

a. **True**

b. **True**

c. **True**

d. **False** – Cholinesterase is an enzyme which breaks down acetylcholine released by the parasympathetic system, terminating its effect

e. **True**

28

Which of these statements are true?

a. Nerve endings in the sympathetic system release noradrenaline (norepinephrine)
b. Nerve endings in the sympathetic system release adrenaline (epinephrine)
c. The adrenal cortex releases adrenaline (epinephrine) and noradrenaline (norepinephrine)
d. There is more than one type of receptor in the sympathetic nervous system
e. There is only one type of receptor in the parasympathetic nervous system

29

Your initial nursing assessment confirms that a patient is in a state of acute anxiety. Which of these statements are true?

a. The patient's feeling of anxiety is a manifestation of the sympathetic nervous system
b. His blood level of adrenaline (epinephrine) will be raised
c. He may be experiencing palpitations
d. His systolic blood pressure will be raised
e. His blood sugar concentration will be lowered

30

Stimulation of the α sympathetic receptors by noradrenaline (norepinephrine) causes:

a. Dilation of the subcutaneous blood vessels
b. Constriction of the pupils
c. A rise in blood pressure
d. A reflex increase in the heart rate
e. A decrease in organ perfusion

28

a. **True**
b. **False** — They release only noradrenaline (norepinephrine)
c. **True** — The renal medulla releases adrenaline (epinephrine) and noradrenaline (norepinephrine), though primarily adrenaline
d. **True** — The sympathetic system contains α receptors, β_1 and β_2 receptors
e. **True**

29

a. **True** — The sensation of anxiety, part of the stress response, is a manifestation of sympathetic stimulation
b. **True** — Adrenaline (epinephrine) is released by the adrenal medulla during the stress response
c. **True** — This results from increased force and rate of cardiac contraction when the sympathetic system is stimulated (β_1 effect) and adrenaline (epinephrine) is released.
d. **True** — Systolic blood pressure rises in response to sympathetic stimulation with increased cardiac output.
e. **False** — Glucose is mobilized and levels of blood sugar increased

30

a. **False** — The subcutaneous blood vessels constrict
b. **False** — The pupils dilate
c. **True**
d. **False** — The heart rate slows reflexly following the rise in blood pressure
e. **True**

31

Adrenaline (epinephrine) can be given by injection in several medical emergencies, particularly anaphylaxis. It is often prescribed as a 1 in 1000 (1 : 1000) solution which contains:

a. 1.0 mg of adrenaline (epinephrine) in 1000 ml
b. 1.0 mg of adrenaline (epinephrine) in 1.0 ml
c. 1.0 g of adrenaline (epinephrine) in 100 ml
d. 1.0 g of adrenaline (epinephrine) in 1000 ml
e. 1.0 μg of adrenaline (epinephrine) in 1000 ml

32

An injection of adrenaline:

a. Stimulates both α and β adrenergic receptors
b. Causes a rise in diastolic blood pressure
c. Causes an increase in heart rate
d. Can cause dangerous cardiac arrhythmias
e. Must be given intravenously

33

You are called to a young patient who is extremely breathless. He tells you that he is asthmatic and explains where to find his salbutamol. Which of these statements are true?

a. Salbutamol is widely prescribed for patients with asthma as it is a potent bronchodilator
b. Salbutamol is a selective β_2 sympathetic agonist
c. Salbutamol should only be used to prevent asthmatic attacks
d. Salbutamol stimulates respiration
e. Salbutamol and other β_2 agonists have replaced adrenaline (epinephrine) and isoprenaline as they have only a minimal stimulating action on the heart

31

a. **False**
b. **True**
c. **False**
d. **True**
e. **False**

32

a. **True**
b. **False** – Raises systolic and lowers diastolic blood pressure
c. **True**
d. **True**
e. **False** – Usually given intramuscularly, intravenous adrenaline (epinephrine) carries the risk of cardiac arrhythmias

33

a. **True**
b. **True**
c. **False** – Salbutamol is probably best used to treat asthmatic attacks when they arise
d. **False**
e. **True** – There was a risk of serious arrhythmias with adrenaline (epinephrine) and isoprenaline

34

In addition to his salbutamol inhaler, which of the following drugs are likely to be prescribed routinely to treat his asthma?

a. A corticosteroid drug
b. Sodium cromoglycate
c. Sodium bicarbonate
d. An antibiotic
e. Slow-release tablets of aminophylline

35

When patients are given salbutamol inhalers, they should be informed of the possible adverse effects, especially if the inhaler is used excessively. These include:

a. Chest pain
b. Tremor
c. Muscle cramps
d. Bronchial infection
e. Palpitations

36

Aminophylline is used in treating asthma:

a. Because it dilates the bronchi
b. It can be given by mouth to prevent asthma attacks
c. Modified release tablets should be chewed before swallowing
d. It can be given intravenously to treat asthma attacks
e. It can cause cardiac arrhythmias

34

a. **True** – Corticosteroids are useful in treating the inflammatory and allergic aspects of asthma and decrease bronchospasm

b. **True** – Sodium cromoglycate is given regularly to prevent asthmatic attacks. It stops mast cells in the bronchi releasing the chemicals which cause bronchospasm

c. **False** – Sodium bicarbonate is used to treat indigestion

d. **False** – Antibiotics would only be prescribed to treat infection

e. **True** – Aminophylline is a bronchodilator. It is sometimes also given to treat an acute asthmatic attack

> **It is important that patients are taught the use of drugs in asthma and to know which are taken regularly to *prevent* attacks and which are used to *relieve* an attack**

35

a. **False**

b. **True**

c. **True**

d. **False**

e. **True** – Although the effect on the heart is minimal

36

a. **True**

b. **True**

c. **False** – They must be swallowed whole

d. **True**

e. **True**

37

Which of the following may precipitate an attack in a patient with asthma?

a. Morphine
b. Aspirin
c. Paracetamol
d. β blockers
e. Exercise

38

A patient with asthma who is starting to use an aerosol inhaler containing salbutamol (a selective β_2 agonist) should be taught:

a. When to use the inhaler
b. How to use the inhaler
c. The possible side-effects
d. When to call the doctor if deterioration occurs
e. How to sterilize the inhaler

39

Adverse effects of the continued use of inhaled steroids for asthma include:

a. Loss of weight
b. A hoarse voice
c. Adrenal suppression with high doses
d. Oral candidiasis
e. Chronic bronchitis

37

a. **False** – Morphine is dangerous if given *during* an attack as it depresses respiration, but it does not cause an asthma attack
b. **True** – And other NSAIAs as well
c. **False**
d. **True** – Can be catastrophic
e. **True**

38

a. **True**
b. **True**
c. **True**
d. **True**
e. **False** – Aerosol inhalers are disposable; however, home nebulizers require special care and maintenance

39

a. **False**
b. **True** – Due to weakness of the laryngeal muscles
c. **True** – This can occur with high doses of inhaled steroids and the patient should be given a card detailing the dose and duration of treatment with steroids
d. **True**
e. **False**

40

In treating status asthmaticus the following should be remembered:

a. Sedation is essential
b. The action of injected corticosteroids may be delayed for some hours
c. Intravenous aminophylline must be given slowly
d. Aminophylline should not be given as an intravenous bolus to those already receiving theophylline by mouth
e. Oxygen (50%) should not be given

41

A young woman is having weekly attacks of migraine and is thus quite disabled. She can be advised to:

a. Look for precipitating factors and avoid them
b. Take ergotamine regularly by mouth
c. Take pizotifen regularly
d. Take a β adrenergic blocking drug regularly
e. Start using an oral contraceptive

42

An attack of migraine classically consists of an aura, followed by headache and vomiting. It can be treated with:

a. Aspirin or paracetamol
b. Metoclopramide
c. A diuretic
d. Sumatriptan
e. Ergotamine

40

a. **False** — It is dangerous
b. **True**
c. **True**
d. **True**
e. **False**

41

a. **True**
b. **False** — Regular ergotamine can cause serious vasoconstriction and make headaches worse
c. **True** — Pizotifen reduces the reactivity of blood vessels and thus prevents migraine. However, it can cause drowsiness and weight gain
d. **True**
e. **False** — Oral contraceptives may precipitate migraines and can be dangerous in certain types of migraine

42

a. **True** — Often adequate
b. **True** — Minimizes vomiting and increases the rate of gastric emptying
c. **False**
d. **True** — Contracts the dilated cerebral vessels
e. **True** — Also a vasoconstrictor, but dosage requires careful regulation

Drugs affecting the cardiovascular system and blood pressure

In the UK cardiovascular disease is the most common cause of death and is also responsible for much acute and chronic illness which can be treated with drugs. In the intensive care and coronary units, nurses will have patients who are critically ill and in whom the precise use of drugs is vital. In the general wards, where patients are less acutely ill, the emphasis will be on relieving such disorders as congestive heart failure and preparing them to return home. In the community, nurses play their part in long-term treatment, educating and advising patients in terms of lifestyle and monitoring their response to treatment and looking out for adverse effects.

In the management of raised blood pressure, nurses in hospital outpatient departments and in the community may be involved.

Many patients are unaware that they are hypertensive until their blood pressure is taken as part of a routine medical check-up or the evidence of long-term hypertension is indicated when their eyes are tested routinely. The news may come as a shock and they may not be willing to comply with medical advice, especially as they may feel perfectly well. Anti-hypertensive drugs may not be necessary if certain changes to their lifestyle are made. However, many patients will still require drug treatment. Nurses can do much to secure adherence to treatment, monitor blood pressure and advise about possible difficulties.

43

The following disorders affecting the heart can be treated with drugs:

a. Cardiac failure
b. Cardiac arrhythmias
c. Cardiac ischaemia
d. Narrowing of the heart valves
e. Congenital heart disease

44

In congestive cardiac failure there is:

a. Poor contraction of the heart muscle
b. A fall in pressure in the veins leading to salt and water retention (oedema)
c. A low cardiac output
d. Inadequate blood supply to the kidneys
e. A decrease in heart rate

45

A retired schoolmistress aged 72 has been diagnosed as having atrial fibrillation and congestive heart failure. During your nursing assessment, what particularly would you look for?

a. Any current drug treatment
b. Pulse rate and rhythm
c. Oedema
d. Shortness of breath
e. Cyanosis

43

a. **True**
b. **True**
c. **True**
d. **False** — Surgical relief is required, although the complications of valve disease (e.g. heart failure) may need drug treatment
e. **False** — Surgical correction is needed, with one rare exception: patent ductus arteriosus in neonates

44

a. **True**
b. **False** — The veins become distended with a rise in pressure
c. **True**
d. **True** — This, with the rise in venous pressure, leads to salt and water retention and oedema
e. **False** — It usually rises

45

a. **True** — A few drugs can exacerbate heart failure (e.g. β blockers)
b. **True** — Arrhythmias, particularly atrial fibrillation, may increase heart failure
c. **True**
d. **True**
e. **True** — Cyanosis may be due to sluggish circulation and poor oxygen uptake in the lungs

46

Which of the following groups of drugs may be given to this patient to improve her heart condition?

a. A diuretic
b. A calcium channel antagonist (nifedipine)
c. Digoxin
d. An angiotensin-converting enzyme (ACE) inhibitor
e. A modified-release potassium preparation

47

It is decided to give this patient digoxin as atrial fibrillation is complicating her congestive heart failure. In your daily observations, which of these suggest to you that the dose of digoxin is too high?

a. Visual disturbances ('yellow vision')
b. Constipation
c. Coupled beats
d. Slight confusion
e. Anorexia

48

You consider that her condition is improving because:

a. Her heart rate has dropped to 65/minute, measured at the apex
b. She has had a diuresis
c. Her weight is dropping
d. Her visitors say she is more like her old self
e. She is less short of breath

46

a. **True** – To relieve oedema and congestion
b. **False** – It might depress cardiac function
c. **True** – By depressing conduction in the AV node it would lower the ventricular rate and make it contract more powerfully and efficiently
d. **True** – By suppressing angiotensin/renin activity it reduces salt and water retention, and by arterial dilation reduces the work of the heart
e. **True** – Could replace potassium loss induced by the diuretic. Potassium loss increases digoxin toxicity. Potassium should not be combined with an ACE inhibitor

47

a. **True**
b. **False**
c. **True** – Due to an overexcitable ventricle causing ectopic beats
d. **True**
e. **True**

48

a. **True** – Largely due to digoxin; if it falls below 55/minute the dose of digoxin should be reduced
b. **True**
c. **True** – Due to loss of oedema fluid
d. **True** – The patient's general condition is a good indicator of her progress
e. **True** – Due to the disappearance of oedema from the lungs and better cardiac function relieving congestion

49

Thiazide diuretics given by mouth are often used in treating congestive cardiac failure. However, they have certain disadvantages:

a. They are short-acting and have to be given three times a day
b. They can make diabetes worse
c. They can cause deafness
d. They are not as powerful as loop diuretics (e.g. frusemide)
e. There is no intravenous preparation available

50

You should ensure that this patient is aware of certain facts regarding her congestive heart failure when she is due to return home:

a. She will require drugs for the rest of her life
b. She should avoid all exercise
c. She should seek advice before starting a new drug
d. Should she experience nausea, she should stop all drugs
e. She must regularly visit her family doctor or medical outpatient department

51

The duration of action of a diuretic is important when designing a drug regimen in order to prevent the diuresis occurring at awkward times (e.g. the middle of the night). Which of these statements are true?

a. Thiazide diuretics usually act for about 12 hours, but vary between preparations
b. Intravenous frusemide acts for about 10 hours
c. Intravenous frusemide acts within half an hour
d. Frusemide given by mouth acts for 24 hours
e. Frusemide given by mouth acts for 6 hours

49

a. **False** – Once a day is the usual dosage
b. **True**
c. **False**
d. **True**
e. **True**

50

a. **True**
b. **False** – Moderate exercise within her tolerance is beneficial
c. **True** – Interaction between her current drug treatment and a new drug is possible and could be dangerous (e.g. NSAIAs reduce the efficacy of diuretics)
d. **False** – Nausea is a side-effect of digoxin and the dose will need to be reduced
e. **True**

51

a. **True**
b. **False** – Usually about 3 hours
c. **True**
d. **False**
e. **True** – Thus frusemide *Lasix* (lasts six)

52

A patient with heart failure, who is already taking a diuretic to which he has partially responded, is to take an ACE inhibitor (captopril). He is advised to take the first dose before retiring for the night because:

a. The drug causes sleepiness
b. The drug is better absorbed lying down
c. There may be a postural fall in blood pressure and, thus, fainting
d. The drug is less liable to cause nausea if the patient is asleep
e. The drug is more effective if taken at night

53

Dopamine may be used to treat patients in shock. Which of the following statements are true?

a. It stimulates contraction of the heart
b. In low doses it increases renal blood flow
c. It should not be combined with dobutamine
d. It is given by mouth to treat Parkinson's disease
e. It should be given via a central venous line

54

A patient with a recent myocardial infarct develops ventricular paroxysmal tachycardia. It is decided to treat this with intravenous lignocaine (lidocaine). The initial dose depends on:

a. The weight of the patient
b. The patient's renal function
c. The patient's liver function
d. The patient's heart rate

55

The rate of the subsequent infusion of lignocaine (lidocaine) is largely influenced by:

a. The weight of the patient
b. The presence or absence of heart failure
c. The patient's liver function
d. The initial dose of lignocaine (lidocaine)

52

a. **False**
b. **False**
c. **True** — Usually only with the first dose
d. **False**
e. **False**

53

a. **True**
b. **True** — Helps to maintain renal function
c. **False**
d. **False** — Dopamine is deficient in Parkinson's disease, but does not enter the brain. Levodopa, which does reach the brain, is used
e. **True** — It can cause intense vasoconstriction

54

a. **True** — The initial dose depends on the volume distribution and, therefore, on the patient's weight
b. **False**
c. **False**
d. **False**

55

a. **False**
b. **True**
c. **True** — The rate of infusion must balance the rate of elimination of the drug, which is eliminated by the liver. Heart failure may reduce liver function
d. **False**

56

A patient is receiving intravenous lignocaine (lidocaine) for paroxysmal tachycardia following a myocardial infarct. What observations are particularly important in this context?

a. Cardiac rate and rhythm
b. Respiratory status
c. Blood pressure
d. Bowel actions
e. Level of consciousness

57

Amiodarone is given for various cardiac arrhythmias. Which of the following are correct?

a. It contains iodine and may be responsible for disturbances of the thyroid function
b. If given intravenously it must be injected slowly via a central venous line
c. Renal function tests must be performed every 6 months as it may cause renal failure
d. Dyspnoea and cough may indicate developing pneumonitis
e. It is rapidly excreted

58

Essential hypertension is a common disorder. In general practice nurses may play an important part in its management. Which is true?

a. It is due to raised cardiac output
b. It is caused by raised peripheral vascular resistance
c. It results from salt and water retention
d. It runs in families
e. It does not require treatment in patients over 60 years of age

56

a. **True** – Lignocaine (lidocaine) can cause bradycardia
b. **True** – Respiratory depression may be a problem
c. **True** – The blood pressure may fall
d. **False**
e. **True**

57

a. **True** – Thyroid function tests should be performed regularly
b. **True** – It is irritant to the vein and may cause hypotension if injected quickly
c. **False**
d. **True** – Chest radiographs should be performed regularly
e. **False** – It is eliminated very slowly

58

a. **False** – But lowering cardiac output reduces blood pressure
b. **True** – Due to narrowing of the arterioles
c. **False** – This can raise blood pressure, but is not found in essential hypertension. Reduced salt intake does, however, lower blood pressure in hypertension
d. **True**
e. **False** – There is considerable benefit up to at least 75 years of age

59

Treating hypertension by lowering the blood pressure:

a. Reduces the risk of stroke
b. Prevents Alzheimer's disease
c. Reduces the risk of heart failure
d. Relieves depression
e. Slows the progression of renal failure

60

The following drugs used to treat hypertension will lower blood pressure:

a. Calcium channel antagonists, by dilating arterioles
b. β Blockers, by a central sedative effect
c. ACE inhibitors, by dilating arterioles and increasing salt and water excretion
d. Thiazide diuretics, by reducing cardiac output
e. Sympathetic blocking drugs, by slowing the pulse

61

A 50-year-old business executive being treated for hypertension with a β blocker may report:

a. Cold hands
b. Palpitations
c. Lack of energy
d. Diarrhoea
e. Difficulty with micturition

59

a. **True** – This is a major benefit of treatment
b. **False**
c. **True**
d. **False**
e. **True**

60

a. **True**
b. **False** – Reduces cardiac output; other mechanisms are probably involved
c. **True**
d. **False** – Increases salt loss and has some vasodilating action
e. **False** – By arteriole dilation

61

a. **True** – β Blockers should not be given to patients with peripheral vascular disease
b. **False**
c. **True**
d. **False**
e. **False**

62

Which of the following statements are true?

a. ACE inhibitors should not be given to treat hypertension of pregnancy
b. Calcium channel blockers should not be given to elderly patients with hypertension
c. β Adrenergic blockers should not be given to patients with asthma
d. Methyldopa is contraindicated in pregnancy
e. Intravenous sodium nitroprusside is very useful in lowering a dangerously raised blood pressure

63

Thiazide diuretics are frequently used to treat essential hypertension. Which of the following are true?

a. They act by lowering peripheral vascular resistance
b. A large dose is usually required
c. They may cause impotence
d. They can be combined with a β blocker
e. They should always be combined with supplementary potassium

64

You are a general practice nurse. What advice about adverse effects would you offer to a patient with hypertension who is starting treatment?

a. Thiazide diuretics can cause attacks of gout
b. ACE inhibitors can cause a cough
c. β Blockers can cause nightmares
d. Calcium channel antagonists can cause cold hands and feet
e. Sympathetic blocking drugs can cause changes in taste

62

a. **True** – Damages the fetus
b. **False**
c. **True** – May cause a severe attack of asthma
d. **False** – It is widely used for hypertension in pregnancy
e. **True** – Requires full monitoring

63

a. **True**
b. **False** – A small dose is effective
c. **True** – About 20% of men
d. **True** – A frequently used combination
e. **False** – Potassium deficiency is very rare if a small dose is used

64

a. **True** – They reduce the excretion of uric acid
b. **True** – Due to the inhibition of breakdown of certain substances
c. **True**
d. **False** – Can, however, cause ankle swelling
e. **False** – This occurs with ACE inhibitors

65

An elderly patient in an old people's home is being treated for hypertension and develops swelling of the ankles. This may be due to:

a. Sitting in a chair all day with the legs dependent
b. Treatment with nifedipine (a calcium channel blocker)
c. Heart failure
d. Treatment with a diuretic
e. Treatment with an ACE inhibitor

66

Blood pressure can be lowered by non-drug methods – these include:

a. Reduction of weight to the ideal level
b. Stopping smoking
c. Lowering salt intake
d. Increasing alcohol consumption
e. Regular exercise

67

When taking the blood pressure of a patient with hypertension who is receiving treatment, you should:

a. Always use the left arm
b. Allow the patient to rest for 5 minutes before taking the blood pressure
c. Record the diastolic pressure as the pressure when all sounds disappear
d. Only take the blood pressure more than 1 hour after a meal
e. Allow nervous patients to take their own blood pressure at home to help reduce their anxiety

65

a. **True**
b. **True** – Probably due to vasodilation
c. **True**
d. **False**
e. **False**

66

a. **True**
b. **False** – Reduces the risk of vascular complications but does not lower blood pressure
c. **True**
d. **False** – Excess alcohol increases blood pressure
e. **True**

67

a. **False** – Usually the right arm is used
b. **True** – Hurrying to keep an appointment may cause a transient rise in blood pressure
c. **True**
d. **False**
e. **True** – Some patients become anxious, which increases their blood pressure (white coat hypertension) and gives an inaccurate impression of their day to day pressures

Anticoagulants and thrombolytic agents

Arterial and venous thrombotic diseases are major causes of death and disability and drugs are important in their treatment and prevention. These diseases are not identical, either in their clinical features or in the underlying processes involved. Their management also differs.

Patients with acute episodes are usually treated in acute units in hospital, but are followed up as outpatients.

Modification of lifestyle and the use of drugs is becoming increasingly important in prevention. The control of symptoms (e.g. anginal pain) is still an important aspect of treatment and requires the correct use of the available drugs.

68

A 56-year-old man is admitted with an acute myocardial infarct (coronary thrombosis). Which of these drugs will probably be used?

a. A thrombolytic agent
b. A calcium channel antagonist
c. An opioid analgesic
d. A phenothiazine anti–emetic
e. Adrenaline

69

Heparin:

a. Is usually given intravenously by a pump
b. Can be given subcutaneously to prevent venous thrombosis
c. Takes about 12 hours to become effective
d. Subcutaneous injection must be given into the buttock
e. Can be used in pregnancy

70

Streptokinase is a thrombolytic agent used in treating coronary thrombosis. Which of these statements are correct?

a. It converts plasminogen in the blood to plasmin, which breaks down the clot (thrombus)
b. It is given by intramuscular injection
c. It is ineffective if given more than 24 hours after the thrombosis occurred
d. Vascular invasive procedures should be avoided, if possible, before and during treatment
e. It should not be combined with aspirin in treating a recent coronary thrombosis

68

a. **True**
b. **False** – It may depress cardiac function
c. **True** – Usually morphine or diamorphine
d. **True** – To prevent vomiting due to the opioid
e. **False** – Unless there is a cardiac arrest

69

a. **True**
b. **True**
c. **False** – Rapid action
d. **False** – Usually into the abdominal wall
e. **True**

70

a. **True**
b. **False** – Given intravenously
c. **True** – The earlier the better
d. **True**
e. **False** – Results are improved if it is combined with aspirin

71

Aspirin prevents arterial thrombosis by:

a. Inhibiting clotting factors
b. Preventing inflammation of the walls of arteries
c. Reducing the number of platelets in the circulation
d. Preventing platelet clumping
e. Preventing arterial spasm

72

Which of the following patients may be advised to take aspirin regularly?

a. A patient with uncomplicated hypertension
b. A patient who has had a transient ischaemic attack
c. A healthy 55-year-old man
d. A patient with unstable angina
e. A patient who has had a venous thrombosis in the leg

73

A patient is leaving hospital after an uneventful recovery from a small myocardial infarct (coronary thrombosis) 2 weeks previously. He has no symptoms, but is asthmatic. What advice would you offer?

a. Bed rest for 2 weeks
b. Give up smoking
c. Reduce weight if raised
d. Take a β adrenergic blocker regularly
e. Take regular glyceryl trinitrate

71

a. **False**
b. **False**
c. **False**
d. **True**
e. **False**

72

a. **False**
b. **True**
c. **False**
d. **True**
e. **False**

73

a. **False** — A graded return to activity is indicated
b. **True**
c. **True**
d. **False** — β Blockers are often advised in these circumstances, but are contraindicated in a patient with asthma
e. **False** — If he has no angina, he would not require this drug

74

Warfarin is widely used as an anticoagulant for venous thrombosis. Which of the following statements are true?

a. Warfarin takes about 2 weeks to become effective
b. The bleeding time is used to measure the effect of warfarin and to control the dosage
c. Warfarin can only be given by mouth
d. Warfarin can cause fetal abnormalities if given in the first 3 months of pregnancy
e. Warfarin can only be given to inpatients in hospital

75

You are teaching a patient about the use of warfarin. You particularly stress that:

a. Overdose is dangerous, causing bleeding
b. Warfarin should be given with food
c. Warfarin should be given at the same time each day
d. Medical advice should be sought before starting or stopping an additional drug as interactions are common
e. A blood sample will be required daily to control dosage

76

Warfarin is contraindicated in:

a. Patients with an active peptic ulcer
b. Patients with valvular heart disease
c. Patients with uncontrolled severe hypertension
d. Patients with severe liver disease
e. Severe renal disease

74

a. **False** – It takes about 3 days
b. **False** – The prothrombin time is used
c. **True**
d. **True**
e. **False** – Many people are treated as outpatients after initial stabilization in hospital

75

a. **True**
b. **False** – Not to be given with food – given alone
c. **True**
d. **True**
e. **False** – When patients are stabilized on a dose, checks are only needed weekly, or even less often

76

a. **True**
b. **False** – But should not be used in patients with infective endocarditis
c. **True** – Risk of a stroke
d. **True**
e. **True**

77

The laboratory reports that a patient taking warfarin has an International Normalised Ratio (INR) of 5.0. There is no evidence of bleeding

a. The INR is the bleeding time divided by the dose of warfarin
b. The INR is the prothrombin time of the patient divided by the normal prothrombin time
c. You should stop the warfarin
d. You should inform a doctor
e. You should repeat the INR measurement the next day

78

The nitrate group of drugs relieves the pain of angina of effort:

a. By slowing the heart rate
b. By dilating the coronary arteries
c. By depressing the contractility of heart muscle
d. By dilating the veins and reducing the cardiac filling pressure
e. By improving oxygenation of the blood

79

When teaching patients how to use glyceryl trinitrate tablets for angina, which statements are true?

a. You must not use the drug more than twice daily
b. Glyceryl trinitrate tablets lose efficacy after being kept for 2 months
c. Tablets of glyceryl trinitrate must be chewed or sucked – if swallowed they are ineffective
d. Glyceryl trinitrate is most effective if used prophylactically before situations which cause anginal pain
e. The tablets take about half an hour to work

77

a. **False**
b. **True**
c. **True**
d. **True**
e. **True**

78

a. **False**
b. **True** – Thus increasing blood supply to the heart muscle
c. **False**
d. **True** – This reduces the work of the heart
e. **False**

79

a. **False** – Take as frequently as required
b. **True** – Should be kept in a closed light-proof container
c. **True** – If swallowed the drug is rapidly broken down as it passes through the liver
d. **True**
e. **False** – It acts in a few minutes

80

Which of these drugs are given *regularly* to prevent attacks of angina of effort?

a. ACE inhibitors
b. β Blockers
c. Digitalis
d. Calcium channel antagonists (e.g. nifedipine)
e. Isosorbide mononitrate

80

a. **False**
b. **True** – Decreases the work of the heart
c. **False**
d. **True** – Dilates the coronary artery
e. **True** – Long-acting nitrate: a vasodilator

Drugs affecting the alimentary tract

In recent years there have been considerable changes in both the investigation and management of gastrointestinal diseases. In particular, the treatment of peptic ulcers has changed with the recognition that this disorder can be effectively treated with drugs. This section explores areas where new approaches are being taken. Care has also been taken to include the less glamorous, but extremely important, topics such as mouth care and bowel management, which have traditionally been nursing responsibilities. The section also considers the management of patients with viral hepatitis and the precautions that health professionals, who have a high risk of exposure to infection, need to employ to ensure their own safety.

81

Part of a patient's nursing assessment includes the inspection of oral hygiene. Which of the following require action?

a. A thick, white coating to the roof of the mouth and over the tongue
b. A generally dry, coated mouth cavity
c. A small ulcer on the tip of the tongue
d. A long, yellow, fang-like molar
e. Evidence of dental plaque

82

An elderly woman reports a burning pain on swallowing and bending forward. She is admitted for endoscopy and her drug history shows that she has been treated by her GP with omeprazole. This drug:

a. Reduces gastric activity by blocking histamine receptors in the stomach (H_2 blocker)
b. May cause gynaecomastia
c. Is more effective than cimetidine in reducing gastric acidity
d. Prolonged use leads to carcinoma of the stomach
e. Is particularly useful in reflux oesophagitis

83

Duodenal ulcers are associated with infection of the pyloric region with *Helicobacter pylori*. Which of the following may be used in combination to eradicate the infection?

a. Bismuth chelate (De Nol)
b. Metronidazole
c. Magnesium trisilicate
d. Clarithromycin
e. Sucralfate

81

a. **True** – This suggests *Candida*, a fungal infection particularly likely to occur in debilitated patients. Treatment is with nystatin or amphotericin lozenges

b. **True** – This indicates dehydration, which must be treated at once

c. **False** – Apthous ulcers are small, painful and often recurrent ulcers, common among healthy people. The cause is unknown and no treatment has been found to be really effective, though local hydrocortisone is sometimes used

d. **True** – Many elderly people need dental treatment and a dental consultation should be sought

e. **True** – Dental plaque may lead to serious infection, especially if the oral cavity becomes dry due to reduced salivation (effect of anaesthesia). Attention to oral hygiene is important

82

a. **False** – It inhibits the proton pump in the stomach lining, which produces acid

b. **False** – Cimetidine has this effect

c. **True**

d. **False** – Previously a worry, but now disproved

e. **True**

83

a. **True**

b. **True**

c. **False**

d. **True**

e. **False**

Various combinations are used and are useful in healing the ulcer and preventing relapse

84

Cimetidine, which is commonly used to treat peptic ulcers:

a. Reduces acidity by blocking H_2 receptors in the stomach
b. Usually relieves the pain of duodenal ulcers after 1 week of treatment
c. When the ulcer has healed, relapse is uncommon
d. May rarely cause impotence
e. Can interact with other drugs

85

A 45-year-old bus driver has had his duodenal ulcer healed by *Helicobacter* eradication. To prevent recurrence or complications you advise him:

a. To avoid aspirin
b. To avoid paracetamol
c. To give up smoking
d. To lose weight
e. To reduce his heavy drinking

86

In the nursing assessment of patients, questions often arise as to the management of constipation. Which of the following are true?

a. Liquid paraffin is the best purgative for children
b. Magnesium sulphate (Epsom salts) should be taken before retiring
c. Senna relieves constipation by stimulating the large bowel and takes about 8 hours to act
d. Co-danthramer is an effective purgative, but its use is restricted by worrying side-effects (evidence of carcinogenicity in animals)
e. Bulk purges are most effective if combined with a high fluid intake

84

a. **True**
b. **True**
c. **False** – Relapse within a year is common after treatment with H_2 blockers
d. **True**
e. **True** – Can reduce the elimination of some drugs (e.g. warfarin, phenytoin)

85

a. **True** – Aspirin and other NSAIAs exacerbate ulceration
b. **False**
c. **True**
d. **False** – Will not affect his ulcer
e. **True**

86

a. **False** – Messy and may be inhaled, or may prevent the absorption of vitamins A, D and K
b. **False** – It acts rapidly and is usually given in the morning
c. **True**
d. **True** – Usually reserved for those with drug-induced constipation (e.g. morphine in patients with a terminal illness)
e. **True**

87

Lactulose is frequently given to elderly patients for the treatment of constipation:

a. It is broken down in the bowel and acts as a mild irritant and osmotic purge
b. It can cause flatulence and distension
c. It acts within 12 hours
d. It is useful in liver disease to reduce the absorption of toxins
e. It is usually given in tablet form

88

A young accountant with persistent severe diarrhoea containing blood has been diagnosed as having ulcerative colitis:

a. Codeine should be used to control the diarrhoea
b. Corticosteroids, either locally or systemically, are effective in curing the colitis
c. Amoxycillin is given to reduce bowel infection
d. After recovery, sulphasalazine may be given to prevent relapses
e. Sulphasalazine can cause serious rashes

89

Loperamide is frequently used in treating diarrhoea:

a. It relieves diarrhoea by sterilizing the bowel
b. It decreases colonic activity
c. In severe diarrhoea, it should be combined with the replacement of fluid and electrolyte loss
d. It can be given as an enema
e. It has a central depressant action

87

a. **True**
b. **True**
c. **False** – Takes several days
d. **True**
e. **False** – It is usually given as a liquid medicine

88

a. **False** – It can cause dangerous bowel distension
b. **True**
c. **False**
d. **True**
e. **True**

89

a. **False**
b. **True**
c. **True**
d. **False**
e. **False**

90

Viral hepatitis B can be serious as it may occasionally lead to chronic liver disease. Nurses may be at special risk owing to their contact with patients:

a. It can be caused by needle-stick injuries
b. It can be caused by the infusion of contaminated blood products
c. It can be transmitted by droplet infection
d. A protective vaccine is available
e. It can be treated, if necessary, with interferons

91

An elderly hypochondriac is receiving multiple drugs. Which of these drugs could have caused his jaundice, particularly in overdose?

a. Lithium
b. Morphine
c. Paracetamol
d. Fucidin
e. Chlorpromazine

90

a. **True**
b. **True**
c. **False**
d. **True**
e. **True** – About 90% of those with hepatitis B recover completely. However, a few develop chronic active hepatitis with progressive liver damage and this group of patients may be treated with interferons.

91

a. **False**
b. **False**
c. **True**
d. **True**
e. **True**

Emetics and anti-emetics

Nausea and vomiting are among the most distressing of symptoms experienced by patients. To control nausea and vomiting nurses need to understand the physiological control mechanisms and how the patient responds to the emetogenic stimulus to be able to administer anti-emetic drugs at times and in doses which will achieve the maximum effect.

92

Nausea and vomiting are associated with many disorders and may also be induced by certain drugs, including:

a. Morphine
b. Levodopa
c. Cimetidine
d. Corticosteroids
e. Estrogens

93

Certain substances in the brain are concerned with vomiting. These include:

a. Noradrenaline (norepinephrine)
b. Dopamine
c. Serotonin (5HT)
d. Acetylcholine
e. GABA

94

To control vomiting:

a. A patient receiving opioids is given prochlorperazine
b. A patient prone to travel sickness is given pyridoxine
c. A patient with migraine-associated vomiting is given metoclopramide
d. A woman vomiting in early pregnancy is given hyoscine
e. A patient with cancer, receiving cisplatin which is very emetic, is given ondansetron

95

Metoclopramide is a useful anti-emetic:

a. It acts by blocking dopamine receptors
b. It increases the rate of gastric emptying
c. In elderly patients it often causes spasm of the muscles of the face and neck
d. It is used in reflux oesophagitis to keep the oesophagus empty
e. It can only be given by injection

92

a. **True**
b. **True**
c. **False**
d. **False**
e. **True**

93

a. **False**
b. **True**
c. **True**
d. **True**
e. **False**

Most anti-emetics work by blocking the effect of these substances

94

a. **True** – Prochlorperazine blocks receptors activated by opioids
b. **False** – Hyoscine or an antihistamine is used
c. **True**
d. **False** – Ineffective and possibly dangerous
e. **True** – It blocks 5HT receptors which are stimulated by cisplatin

95

a. **True**
b. **True**
c. **False** – This occurs more commonly in young patients
d. **True**
e. **False** – Usually given by mouth

Analgesics

Effective pain control is one of the most vital aims of patient care. Much depends on careful assessment so that the appropriate analgesic drug is selected and administered, modifying the dose schedule to meet the needs of the patient. The long-term use of analgesics may be associated with adverse effects, which can be avoided or reduced by taking the appropriate steps. It is impossible to over-emphasize the role of patient education and support in determining the effectiveness of strategies to relieve pain. These activities require a sound knowledge of clinical pharmacology and excellent communication skills.

In hospital, the relief of pain in both surgical and medical care involves nurses daily. The control of long-term pain, particularly in oncology and palliative care units, has become a speciality requiring considerable expertise. Most hospitals now have a pain control team. Nurses, particularly those in community health care, should also be aware of the many analgesics available 'over the counter' without prescription.

96

Analgesics may relieve pain by:

a. Inducing sleepiness
b. Reducing inflammation or other changes at painful sites
c. Blocking conduction in the peripheral nerves
d. Stimulating the release of inhibitors in the brain
e. Stimulating receptors in the brain and spinal cord which inhibit pain appreciation

97

A 40-year-old publican has cirrhosis of the liver. He has severe pain and requires morphine. Particular care with dosage is needed because:

a. Absorption of the drug into the circulation will be reduced
b. The ability of his liver to eliminate the drug will be impaired
c. Part of the portal circulation will bypass the liver
d. Liver damage may be further increased
e. Morphine will penetrate more readily into the brain

98

The patient's relatives have heard that morphine is dangerous and are worried. You explain to them that it is the drug of choice for him, but that it has a number of side-effects:

a. It depresses respiration in overdose
b. It should be used with care in those with chronic bronchitis
c. It causes fits
d. It causes constipation
e. He will become dependent on it

96

a. **False**
b. **True** – The mode of action of NSAIAs
c. **True** – The mode of action of local anaesthetics
d. **False**
e. **True** – The mode of action of opioids

97

a. **False**
b. **True**
c. **True**
d. **False**
e. **False**

98

a. **True**
b. **True** – Due to respiratory depression
c. **False**
d. **True** – If used regularly, an aperient will be required
e. **False** – Dependence is rare if it is given for severe pain of short duration

99

The following are true of morphine:

a. Given by mouth, it is more effective in a single dose than with repeated doses
b. It causes nausea in about 15% of patients receiving it
c. It should be avoided in patients with acute heart failure
d. It is available as a slow-release oral preparation
e. Its actions are enhanced in patients with renal failure

100

A titled lady has terminal cancer. She is aware of the diagnosis and has participated in her own care. She is interested in pain relief, but has become rather muddled and asks you to clarify these points:

a. NSAIAs are useless in her condition
b. If she takes morphine solution by mouth, it will be needed every 12 hours
c. High doses of morphine will always be needed
d. The morphine will render her unable to carry on a reasonable conversation
e. Morphine solution will expire after storage for 6 months

101

Which of the following statements are correct?

a. Pethidine is used in the later stages of labour
b. Methadone is used to treat morphine overdose
c. Codeine is used to treat diarrhoea
d. Naloxone is used in patients with terminal cancer
e. Buprenorphine can be used for moderately severe pain

99

a. **False** – Repeated dosing is more effective because of the accumulation of an active breakdown product
b. **True**
c. **False** – It may be part of the management of this disorder
d. **True**
e. **True**

100

a. **False** – They are sometimes very effective, especially for bone pain
b. **False** – It is usually only effective for 4–6 hours
c. **False**
d. **False** – Not necessarily so
e. **False** – Three months

101

a. **True** – Because it is short-acting
b. **False** – Used for replacement therapy in patients with opioid dependence
c. **True**
d. **False** – Used in opioid overdose because it blocks the effect of opioids
e. **True**

Note: It is now considered that pethidine (a) is not very effective in the later stages of labour.

102

Minor analgesic drugs are frequently used in hospital and at home. Your patient has read an article about aspirin and asks you to confirm these points:

a. The analgesic action of aspirin lasts about 4 hours
b. Soluble aspirin does not produce gastric bleeding
c. Children under 14 years should not be given aspirin
d. Paracetamol is safe for those with peptic ulceration
e. Co-proxamol (Distalgesic) is a very safe analgesic

103

Non-steroidal anti-inflammatory agents are widely used for rheumatoid arthritis and many minor aches and pains:

a. They block the action of cyclo-oxygenase and thus suppress the formation of prostaglandins which are responsible for the inflammation and pain
b. They depress conduction in pain pathways in the spinal cord
c. They can cause indigestion and gastric bleeding
d. They can all be purchased 'over the counter' without prescription
e. They antagonize the action of diuretics and hypotensive drugs

104

A middle-aged woman has suffered from rheumatoid arthritis for many years. The following drugs are likely to have been used in her treatment:

a. NSAIAs will have been the initial treatment
b. NSAIAs are all equally liable to have adverse effects
c. Disease-modifying drugs such as gold were used when NSAIAs were not successful
d. Disease-modifying drugs are useful because of their rapid action
e. Corticosteroids

102

a. **True**

b. **False**

c. **True** – Aspirin rarely causes a dangerous reaction. Paracetamol should be used

d. **True**

e. **False** – It is a combination of paracetamol and dextropropoxyphene and can be dangerous with fairly minor overdose

103

a. **True**

b. **False**

c. **True**

d. **False** – Only ibuprofen does not require a doctor's prescription

e. **True**

104

a. **True** – This is likely, though changes are being made to drug regimens

b. **False** – Ibuprofen appears to be safer, but perhaps less effective

c. **True**

d. **False** – Their therapeutic effect may be delayed for a month or two

e. **False** – Corticosteroids are not used routinely in the treatment of rheumatoid arthritis, except in special circumstances

105

She attends the clinic at monthly intervals. Which disease-modifying drugs might she be given?

a. Sulphasalazine
b. Gold
c. Probenecid
d. Indomethacin
e. Methotrexate

106

In fact, she was being treated with penicillamine. Which tests should be performed regularly?

a. ECG
b. Urine test for protein
c. Liver function tests
d. Blood count
e. Chest radiograph

107

A brilliant, but somewhat choleric, cleric has an acute episode of gout. Which of the following will the GP prescribe to relieve his symptoms?

a. Allopurinol
b. Colchicine
c. An NSAIA
d. A high fluid intake
e. A thiazide diuretic

105

a. **True**
b. **True**
c. **False** – Used in gout to increase the excretion of uric acid
d. **False** – It is an NSAIA
e. **True**

106

a. **False**
b. **True** – Proteinuria may develop
c. **False**
d. **True** – Depression of the blood count, including platelets, is an adverse effect.
e. **False**

107

a. **False** – It is used to prevent attacks
b. **True** – Though an NSAIA is more usual
c. **True**
d. **False** – Not essential unless the patient is dehydrated, but necessary if a uricosuric drug is used to prevent attacks
e. **False** – It may cause an attack of gout

Hypnotic drugs

In recent years there has been a move away from the previously widespread and sometimes indiscriminate use of hypnotic drugs. It is now apparent that with careful patient assessment and management such drugs are generally unnecessary, especially as they become less effective with continued use and withdrawal symptoms may cause problems. However, large numbers of patients in hospital and the community report sleeping difficulties. Elderly people are particularly likely to experience problems sleeping and may expect or request drugs. Before hypnotic drugs are given it is important to establish whether they are really necessary through careful assessment, as other nursing strategies may in the long term be more effective and less likely to result in dependence.

108

A 68-year-old retired railwayman tells you that he rarely has a good night's sleep. Possible causes are:

a. Taking a glass of milk before retiring
b. Taking two cups of coffee after dinner
c. Depression
d. Heart failure
e. Exercise during the day

109

Eventually a benzodiazepine is prescribed to help him to sleep. These drugs, which are still commonly (perhaps too commonly) prescribed, have a number of adverse effects:

a. They have a marked depressant effect on respiration
b. Repeated use can lead to dependence and withdrawal symptoms
c. They may cause nausea
d. Once stopped, rebound insomnia can occur
e. Some may cause 'hang over' effects (drowsiness) into the next day

110

A 72-year-old retired soldier is under the care of the community psychiatric nurse. He lives alone and has a marked fondness for alcohol. Periodically he decides to reduce his intake, but experiences agitation and insomnia. Chlormethiazole is suggested as a good choice of sedative for him:

a. It is effective in reducing the symptoms associated with alcohol withdrawal
b. It is not potentially addictive
c. It is safe, even in overdose
d. It has few side-effects, but can cause nasal congestion
e. It has some antiepileptic action

108

a. **False** – May help sleep in some people
b. **True**
c. **True**
d. **True**
e. **False** – Regular exercise during the day helps sleep at night

109

a. **False**
b. **True** – Should only be used for short periods (up to 2 weeks)
c. **False**
d. **True**
e. **True** – Particularly in elderly patients

110

a. **True**
b. **False** – Dependence on alcohol may change to dependence on chlormethiazole
c. **False** – Central depression can occur and it is important that the patient does not overdose or combine it with alcohol. Particular care is needed if it is given by intravenous infusion to sedate seriously disturbed patients
d. **True**
e. **True** – It can be given intravenously to control status epilepticus

111

Nurses working in the community may be asked about the use of promethazine as a hypnotic drug:

a. It is available without prescription
b. It can be used to treat children
c. There is no 'hang over' effect the next morning
d. It is an antihistamine and can be used systemically for skin irritation
e. It is also a mild analgesic

111

a. **True**
b. **True** – Although the unnecessary use of hypnotic drugs in children should be discouraged
c. **False** – Sedation may persist into the next day
d. **True**
e. **False**

Drugs used in anaesthesia

All nurses need to be regularly updated in cardiopulmonary resuscitation procedures and to maintain an up to date knowledge of the drugs likely to be used during cardiac or respiratory arrest.

The role of the nurse anaesthetist is now well established in the USA and, given that innovations in the delivery of nursing and medical care often travel from the USA to the UK, it follows that nurses in the UK may in future need to increase the breadth and depth of their knowledge of anaesthetic drugs. It is probable that only a few specialist and highly qualified nurses will become actively involved in the administration of anaesthesia, but the role of nurses in pre- and post-operative care is well established. They need to be able to observe and monitor patients for the effects of drugs administered during the peri-operative period and to explain their effects to patients and their families, preferably before the operation or investigation.

As the role of the nurse practitioner develops, increasing numbers of hospital and community-based nurses working in nurse-led units will develop high levels of expertise in performing particular procedures or investigations. In many cases this will entail the administration of local anaesthesia by the nurse.

112

A 56-year-old schoolmistress is to have a lumpectomy for carcinoma of the breast and she is very anxious about it. What means are available to reduce her anxiety:

a. Premedication with atropine
b. Premedication with morphine
c. Listening to the patient's worries
d. Premedication with β blockers
e. Premedication with diazepam

113

Atropine is frequently used for premedication:

a. It is a muscle relaxant
b. It increases the pulse rate
c. It reduces salivary secretion
d. It prevents post-operative urinary retention
e. It may cause blurring of vision

114

The muscle relaxant suxamethonium is often combined with a general anaesthetic:

a. To facilitate intubation of the trachea
b. During surgery, to facilitate the closing of the abdomen
c. In the post-operative period, it may produce muscle pains
d. Its action is reversed by neostigmine
e. In the treatment of myasthenia gravis

115

Local anaesthetics block the transmission of impulses along nerves. This can be achieved by:

a. Application to mucous membranes or skin
b. Local infiltration of the painful area
c. Injection around local nerves
d. Epidural injection
e. Injection into pain fibres in the spinal cord

112

a. **False** – Atropine has little sedative action
b. **True**
c. **True** – Very important
d. **False** – Although β blockers suppress some aspects of anxiety,
they are not used for this purpose before surgery
e. **True**

113

a. **False**
b. **True** – By blocking the vagus nerve (parasympathetic)
c. **True**
d. **False**
e. **True** – Due to paralysis of accommodation

114

a. **True**
b. **True**
c. **True**
d. **False** – Although this is true of some muscle relaxants
e. **False**

115

a. **True** – For example, Emla cream applied to the skin
b. **True**
c. **True** – For example, mandibular block used in dentistry
d. **True** – For example, the relief of labour pain
e. **False**

116

It is important to calculate the correct dose of a local anaesthetic for a given procedure. Mistakes can occur and local anaesthetics can be dangerous in overdose. A 1% solution contains:

a. 1 g in 100 ml
b. 1 mg in 100 ml
c. 10 mg in 1 ml
d. 1 g in 1 ml
e. 100 mg in 100 ml

117

Pain in the immediate post-operative period may be a cause of:

a. Hyperpyrexia
b. A rise in pulse rate
c. A rise in blood pressure
d. Obstruction of the upper airway
e. Anxiety and restlessness

118

In the control of post-operative pain:

a. It is important to have a flexible programme to keep the patient pain-free, as people vary in their needs
b. Always use an opioid analgesic
c. Use reassurance and explanation
d. The use of oxygen by face mask is useful
e. 'Patient-controlled analgesia' can be very effective

119

During cardiopulmonary resuscitation, drugs may be given:

a. Intravenously
b. Subcutaneously
c. Down an endotracheal tube
d. Intra-osseously
e. Rectally

116

a. **True**
b. **False**
c. **True**
d. **False**
e. **False**

117

a. **False**
b. **True**
c. **True**
d. **False**
e. **True**

118

a. **True**
b. **False** – Opioids are frequently, but not always, necessary
c. **True**
d. **False** – Oxygen has no analgesic properties
e. **True**

119

a. **True** – Preferably via a central line
b. **False** – Absorption is very slow due to lack of circulation to subcutaneous tissue
c. **True** – Rarely used, but atropine and lignocaine (lidocaine) are absorbed by this route
d. **True** – Particularly in children
e. **False** – Too slow

Drugs used in psychiatry

The use of drugs is probably the most important active treatment available for people with psychiatric disorders. The mental health problems most amenable to drug treatment are schizophrenia, affective disorders (depressive and manic states) and psychoneurosis. Although each of these is associated with its own armoury of preferred drugs, some are used to treat more than one disorder. As research progresses it is becoming apparent that schizophrenia and the affective disorders are associated with the malfunction of neurotransmitter substances or their receptors in the brain. Most drugs now used modify the actions of neurotransmitters or their receptors.

A significant proportion of the adult population take drugs intended to help some mental health problem and, while they may be receiving care from specialist nurses, they will often be admitted to general hospital wards or consult a district or practice nurse for some other, unrelated, health problem. The drugs used to treat mental health problems may react with other drugs or foods, so it is important that all nurses have some knowledge of their interactions and mode of action.

120

A farmer reports strange noises and tells the community psychiatric nurse that he cannot sleep at night because a large mouse runs round his bedroom. He also has delusions that somebody is trying to shut him in a blanket chest which stands at the foot of his bed. Phenothiazines have been prescribed for his psychotic state. Which of the following are true of this group of drugs?

a. They block dopamine receptors in the brain
b. They relieve depression
c. They are antipsychotic
d. They are anti-emetic
e. They are antiepileptic

121

The community psychiatric nurse responsible for his management will need to monitor him for which of the following adverse effects caused by the chlorpromazine he is taking?

a. Raised blood pressure
b. Dystonia
c. Jaundice
d. Hiccups
e. Exposure to sun

122

It becomes apparent that his paranoid state will require long-term treatment with phenothiazines, but it seems unlikely that he will take his drugs regularly. The nurse explains that compliance can be improved by giving depot injections. The following information is given to the patient and his family. Which is correct?

a. The injection will be given into the upper arm
b. A small test dose is given to assess his response
c. Only 8 ml will be given at a particular site
d. The effect of the injection will last about 12 weeks
e. As the response is variable, the dose may require adjustment

120

a. **True**
b. **False**
c. **True**
d. **True**
e. **False** — They may provoke fits under certain circumstances

121

a. **False** — Chlorpromazine causes a fall in blood pressure on standing and should therefore be measured standing, as well as lying
b. **True** — Various disorders of movement can occur, including akathisia (inability to remain still)
c. **True**
d. **False** — It is sometimes used to control hiccups
e. **True** — Photosensitivity can occur and a sunscreen is needed

122

a. **False** — The gluteal muscle is used
b. **True**
c. **False** — Usually 2–3 ml
d. **False** — 1–4 weeks
e. **True**

123

Phenothiazines should usually be avoided in patients with:

a. Closed angle glaucoma
b. Epilepsy
c. Parkinson's disease
d. Anxiety
e. Hypertension

124

Schizophrenia:

a. Is largely, but not entirely, due to a disorder of dopamine receptors in the brain
b. Phenothiazine drugs are useful in its management
c. Long-term treatment is not necessary
d. Clozapine is useful for patients who respond poorly to initial treatment
e. Clozapine has no serious side-effects

125

A 64-year-old retired postman has had difficulty in sleeping for some time, he has lost his appetite and has no interest in life. When asked what is wrong, he says he is useless and there is no point in life. Severe endogenous (psychotic) depression of this nature is believed to be caused by a disorder of transmitter substances in the brain. Which may be involved?

a. Acetylcholine
b. Serotonin (5HT)
c. GABA
d. Noradrenaline (norepinephrine)
e. Angiotensin

123

a. **True** — Makes them worse
b. **True** — Makes them worse
c. **True** — Makes them worse
d. **False**
e. **False**

124

a. **True** — But still debated
b. **True**
c. **False** — It is nearly always necessary
d. **True**
e. **False** — It can cause depression of the white cells

125

a. **False**
b. **True**
c. **False**
d. **True**
e. **False**

126

Amitriptyline (tricyclic antidepressant) has been prescribed for a patient. This drug increases the noradrenaline (norepinephrine) and serotonin in the brain and is suitable for an elderly man living alone because:

a. It is safe in overdose
b. It is not addictive
c. Depression will be relieved in a few days
d. It does not produce vomiting
e. It will also help to relieve his symptoms of prostatism

127

When he starts taking amitriptyline, you give him the following information:

a. He must take the tablets three times daily
b. He may experience constipation and a dry mouth
c. He must keep the tablets in a safe place
d. He must consult a doctor or pharmacist before taking any other drugs
e. He should not stop them suddenly

128

His son has read about the new antidepressants (5HT re-uptake inhibitors) and wants to know whether fluoxetine would be better for his father because:

a. It has no serious effects on the heart
b. It is more effective than amitriptyline
c. It improves the appetite
d. It is safer in overdose
e. It is cheaper

126

a. **False** – It is particularly cardiotoxic
b. **True** – Worries about dependence are fairly common
c. **False** – May take up to 6 weeks
d. **True**
e. **False** – It may exacerbate urinary retention

127

a. **False** – Once daily, usually before retiring
b. **True**
c. **True**
d. **True**
e. **True** – They must be tailed off gradually

128

a. **True**
b. **False** – They are equally effective
c. **False** – It can cause nausea
d. **True**
e. **False** – More expensive

129

In your care is a 45-year-old man who is taking a monoamine oxidase (MAO) inhibitor. The following, elicited from his nursing assessment, fills you with alarm:

a. He has a cold and is taking a proprietary remedy
b. For supper he has had a Marmite sandwich and cheese and biscuits
c. He now has a severe headache
d. He often dribbles when excited
e. He is due for premedication with pethidine in half an hour

130

A 40-year-old housewife has bipolar depression and is to start taking lithium. The dose is critical and toxicity can easily occur. You therefore tell her:

a. To take the drug three time a day in small doses
b. To test her urine daily for protein
c. To get her blood level of lithium measured regularly
d. To stop the drug for 1 week every 6 months
e. To carry a card explaining her treatment

131

The following may increase the blood level of lithium and will necessitate alteration of the dose:

a. A β blocker
b. A thiazide diuretic
c. Morphine
d. Penicillin
e. A serious attack of diarrhoea

129

a. **True**   – It may contain a vasoconstricting substance and its action would be greatly enhanced
b. **True**   – Marmite and cheese, and some other articles of diet contain substances which cause a rise in blood pressure when combined with MAO inhibitors
c. **True**   – It has caused a severe rise in blood pressure!
d. **False**
e. **True**   – A serious interaction may occur

130

a. **False**   – Once daily
b. **False**
c. **True**
d. **False**
e. **True**

131

a. **False**
b. **True**
c. **False**
d. **False**
e. **True**   – Due to sodium loss and a corresponding rise in blood lithium levels

132

Adverse effects of lithium include:

a. Thyroid deficiency
b. Confusion
c. Diarrhoea
d. Headaches
e. Weight loss

132

a. **True**
b. **True**
c. **True**
d. **False**
e. **False**

Antiepileptic drugs and drugs used to treat Parkinson's disease

Most patients with epilepsy are managed within the community. They are monitored and receive drugs to abolish seizures either in hospital outpatient departments or via their GP. The aim of treatment is to allow the patient to live as fully and independently as possible. A range of drugs effective in the control of different types of epilepsy is now available. The challenge is to select a drug which will have the optimum efficacy for the individual patient with minimal side-effects. Nurses involved in the care of these patients and their families play an important part in documenting the response to antiepileptic drugs, asking about side-effects and securing adherence to the treatment regimen. Such an undertaking clearly requires both a sound understanding of the different types of epilepsy, the effects of the disorder on individuals and their families and the action of antiepileptic drugs.

Parkinson's disease is a chronic progressive disorder of the nervous system chiefly affecting older people. A number of different drugs may be prescribed to control the symptoms and improve the patient's quality of life. Again, patients can be managed either through a hospital outpatient department, or by their GP. Successful management involves tailoring the treatment regimen to the needs of the individual patient. Practice nurses and nurse specialists employed in hospital clinics are playing an increasingly important part in the care of such patients.

133

A 17-year-old schoolboy has been given a diagnosis of tonic-clonic (grand mal) epilepsy following an episode in which he briefly lost consciousness and fell out of a tree while birdwatching. On questioning, he remembers other episodes when he briefly lost consciousness without warning. Phenytoin is prescribed to prevent further attacks. However, his mother has been told that finding the optimum dose may be difficult. This is because:

a. It is poorly absorbed from the gut
b. It is eliminated slowly (long half-life) and will take about a week to achieve a steady blood concentration
c. Individuals vary as to the rate at which they eliminate phenytoin
d. Phenytoin may interact with other drugs
e. The relationship between dose and blood level is variable (non-linear)

134

He has been told to look out for various side-effects which may be related to taking phenytoin. These include:

a. Tremor
b. Diarrhoea
c. Insomnia
d. Drowsiness
e. Fever/sore throat

135

In spite of efforts to control his epilepsy, including repeated measurement of plasma levels of the drug, he still has fits and it is decided to replace phenytoin with carbamazepine. However, there can be difficulties with this drug:

a. It often requires an increase in the initial dose as the rate of elimination increases with use
b. Children eliminate the drug more slowly than adults, so once daily dosing is adequate
c. It is not so effective as phenytoin in controlling tonic-clonic epilepsy
d. It occasionally causes bone marrow depression
e. It may cause a widespread erythematous rash

133

a. **False** – But can be variable
b. **True**
c. **True**
d. **True**
e. **True**

134

a. **True**
b. **False**
c. **True**
d. **True** – With too large a dose
e. **True** – May indicate depression of blood count

135

a. **True**
b. **False** – Children eliminate the drug more rapidly
c. **False** – They are similar
d. **True**
e. **True**

136

The patient then goes through a rebellious mood and stops taking his carbamazepine tablets. You are the triage nurse in the A & E department of the local hospital when he is admitted in status epilepticus. Emergency action will include:

a. Ensuring the airway remains patent
b. Administering 60% oxygen
c. Giving diazepam intravenously
d. Giving phenytoin intravenously
e. Passing a nasogastric tube

137

A patient with epilepsy, being treated with sodium valproate, is admitted to hospital for a gastrectomy. Before the operation it is necessary to:

a. Measure the blood level of sodium valproate
b. Perform liver function tests
c. Perform a blood count, including platelets
d. Collect a 24-hour urine sample
e. Stop the sodium valproate

138

Patients taking antiepileptic drugs need to be given the following information, depending on their individual circumstances:

a. Treatment of a pregnant woman with antiepileptic drugs sometimes causes fetal abnormalities
b. Carbamazepine and sodium valproate can cause neural tube defects
c. It is possible to withdraw drug treatment for epilepsy if the patient has been free of fits for 5 years
d. A patient diagnosed as epileptic can never drive a car again
e. Only about 30% of patients with tonic-clonic epilepsy are controlled by a single drug

136

a. **True**
b. **True**
c. **True** – Given as Diazemuls, a non-irritant preparation
d. **True** – After initial control, relapse may occur and can be prevented by phenytoin
e. **False** – Place in the lateral semiprone position

137

a. **False** – It is not helpful
b. **True** – Valproate can affect the liver
c. **True** – It can also cause platelet deficiency
d. **False**
e. **False**

138

a. **True**
b. **True**
c. **True** – Withdrawal of drugs must be slow
d. **False**
e. **False** – About 80% are controlled

139

An unmarried mother with four children under 5 years of age rushes into the A & E department, distraught. Her baby has just had a convulsion and feels very hot. When the baby has received treatment you are able to reassure her:

a. Febrile convulsions are common, occurring in about 3% of young children
b. Most children who have a febrile convulsion will only suffer mild epilepsy afterwards
c. If the convulsions recur, they can be controlled by rectal diazepam
d. If the fever occurs at home, the child can be given aspirin
e. Prophylactic ethosuximide can be given to prevent further fits

140

A widower, who has retired from his employment as a miner, has moved to London to live near his daughter. She is concerned as he seems so much slower and she notices that his hands shake. She accompanies him to his GP, who diagnoses Parkinson's disease. She thought he might have a mental problem, and is reassured that Parkinson's disease is a biochemical disorder, amenable to drug treatment:

a. The disease is due to dopamine deficiency in the basal ganglia of the brain
b. Levodopa is used in treatment as it penetrates the brain: dopamine does not
c. Levodopa is converted to dopamine in the brain
d. Levodopa is ineffective in elderly patients
e. Levodopa is usually combined with a decarboxylase inhibitor as this increases elimination

139

a. **True**
b. **False** – Very few develop epilepsy
c. **True**
d. **False** – Paracetamol, not aspirin, should be used to reduce fever
e. **False**

140

a. **True**
b. **True**
c. **True**
d. **False**
e. **False** – The inhibitor decreases the breakdown of levodopa in the tissues, increasing efficacy and reducing adverse effects

141

He is referred to a clinic specializing in the treatment of Parkinson's disease. Levodopa is prescribed and he is warned by the nurse specialist to look out for these side-effects:

a. Postural hypotension (faintness on standing)
b. Nausea
c. Muscle cramps
d. Decreasing efficacy after years of treatment
e. Headaches

142

A number of other drugs may be given to treat Parkinson's disease. Which of the following statements are correct?

a. Selegiline works by preventing the breakdown of levodopa
b. Selegiline may be combined with levodopa when the latter becomes ineffective
c. Bromocriptine can be used as it acts in a similar way to dopamine
d. Anticholinergic drugs (e.g. benzhexol) are prescribed, but adverse effects are troublesome
e. Tremor responds better than rigidity to levodopa

143

A number of drugs are well known for inducing a Parkinson-like state. They include:

a. Tricyclic antidepressants (e.g. amitriptyline)
b. The phenothiazine neuroleptics (e.g. chlorpromazine)
c. The monoamine-oxidase inhibitors
d. The benzodiazepines (e.g. diazepam)
e. Lithium

141

a. **True**
b. **True**
c. **False**
d. **True**
e. **False**

142

a. **True**
b. **True**
c. **True**
d. **True** – Side-effects include dry mouth, constipation and blurred vision
e. **False** – The other way round

143

a. **False**
b. **True**
c. **False**
d. **False**
e. **False**

The endocrine system

Diseases of the endocrine system are common and a wide range of drugs is used to treat them. As hormones play such a vital part in the control of physiological functions, a sound understanding of normal physiology is important when tackling this complex topic.

Probably the most common endocrinological disorder involving nurses is the management of diabetes. Whether in hospital or the community, some nurses will specialize in patients with this disease. They may be required to advise on lifestyle and the use of drugs and also be familiar with the various complications and crises which may occur, acting as mentor and guide to patients and their families.

The use of sex hormones in women, including oral contraceptives and hormone replacement therapy, is widespread and, to some degree, controversial, and again, nurses are involved. We have, therefore, given prominence to these two areas.

Steroid hormones are important drugs with considerable potential for both good and harm, so careful monitoring of the patient is particularly necessary.

Other situations in which drugs are used to modify the action of hormones, including the thyroid, have been included.

144

Before teaching patients, their families or junior colleagues about drugs affecting the endocrine system, it is essential to be clear about the naturally secreted hormones and their effects. Revise briefly the hormones released from the pituitary gland, which controls so much of the endocrine activity in the rest of the body. The following hormones are released from the anterior lobe:

a. Insulin
b. Oxytocin
c. Prolactin
d. Prednisolone
e. Follicle-stimulating hormone

145

A patient who has had a stillbirth has been given bromocriptine to suppress lactation. This drug:

a. Acts on the breast to inhibit milk secretion
b. Reduces prolactin secretion by the pituitary gland
c. Stimulates dopamine receptors
d. Causes nausea and vomiting
e. Is used in the treatment of Parkinson's disease

146

A 40-year-old housewife has been feeling very slow and lethargic. She feels cold and, although she is not eating well, has put on weight. Her doctor recognizes all the signs and symptoms of an underactive thyroid gland (myxoedema) and this is borne out by the results of blood tests. Which of the following information is appropriate?

a. Thyroxine given by mouth is the drug of choice
b. She will need to take tablets once a week
c. She should look out for palpitations and may lose weight when treated
d. She will start with a high dose which will probably be reduced later
e. She should seek medical help if she notices chest pain on exertion (angina of effort)

144

a. **False** – The pancreas
b. **False** – Post-pituitary
c. **True**
d. **False** – A synthetic hormone related to cortisone
e. **True**

145

a. **False**
b. **True**
c. **True**
d. **True**
e. **True**

Cabergoline, a very similar drug, is preferred by many as it is better tolerated and has a longer action

146

a. **True**
b. **False** – Usually given once daily
c. **True**
d. **False** – Start with a low dose and increase slowly until the correct response is achieved
e. **True**

147

A middle-aged man has found his old friend sadly changed. She used to be a pleasant companion, happy to sit and watch the world go by, now she rushes about, becomes excited about nothing and is very argumentative. He persuades her to visit the health centre for a check up where blood tests are performed. They confirm a diagnosis of thyrotoxicosis (hyperactive thyroid gland). Which of the following may be prescribed to control this disorder?

a. Corticosteroids
b. Spironolactone
c. Iodine solution
d. Carbimazole
e. β Adrenergic blockers

148

A patient who has been prescribed prednisolone is told that its therapeutic actions could include:

a. Suppressing inflammation
b. Enhancing immunity
c. Suppressing immunity
d. Treating adrenal deficiency (Addison's disease)
e. Treating some malignant diseases (e.g. lymphomas)

149

Which of the following must he undergo regularly in view of his long-term treatment with corticosteroids (prednisolone)?

a. Measurement of blood pressure
b. Checking the peripheral pulses
c. Testing his urine for glucose
d. Regular inquiry about indigestion
e. Throat swab

147

a. **False**
b. **False**
c. **True** – Only used in the initial stages before surgery
d. **True** – Reduces thyroid hormone secretion
e. **True** – Controls symptoms due to overactivity of the sympathetic nervous system (e.g. tachycardia)

148

a. **True**
b. **False**
c. **True**
d. **False** – Hydrocortisone and fludrocortisone are the preferred drugs
e. **True**

149

a. **True**
b. **False**
c. **True** – Occasionally a diabetic-like state develops
d. **True** – May exacerbate peptic ulcers
e. **False**

150

A man is admitted to hospital with pneumonia. His nursing assessment reveals that he has been taking prednisolone by mouth for several years. What action would be taken?

a. Prednisolone stopped at once
b. Usual dose continued while he is in hospital
c. The dose of prednisolone would be increased
d. The appropriate antibiotic would be given
e. His blood pressure would be monitored

151

He makes a good recovery and is ready to be discharged from hospital. The following points should be emphasized concerning his prednisolone:

a. He should take the main dose before retiring
b. He should not visit his sister while her children have chicken pox
c. Muscular development increases
d. He must not suddenly stop taking his tablets
e. He should always carry a card giving details of his treatment

152

A 10-year-old schoolgirl has just been diagnosed as having type I (insulin-dependent) diabetes. As the specialist nurse responsible for co-ordinating her care and educating her family, you provide the following information concerning the action of insulin:

a. It stimulates the pancreas
b. It increases glucose absorption from the gut
c. It increases insulin uptake by tissues
d. It lowers the plasma glucose concentration
e. It can only be given by injection

150

a. **False**
b. **False**
c. **True** — Corticosteroid dosage must be increased during a severe infection as there is a danger of collapse if a deficiency develops
d. **True**
e. **True**

151

a. **False** — Corticosteroids can cause insomnia
b. **True** — Chicken pox may be a serious disease for him as his immunity will be suppressed by the prednisolone
c. **False**
d. **True** — This would cause collapse with low blood pressure
e. **True**

152

a. **False** — It is secreted by the pancreas
b. **False**
c. **True**
d. **True**
e. **True** — It is broken down in the stomach

153

The girl's mother will require guidance on:

a. Diet
b. Administration of insulin
c. The symptoms and signs of hypoglycaemia
d. The technique of intravenous injection
e. Testing the blood/urine for glucose

154

Her mother has heard about diabetic (ketoacidotic) comas and wants to know how they are treated. You explain that for a patient with hyperglycaemic ketoacidosis:

a. Insulin will be given subcutaneously
b. Soluble insulin will be used
c. Very large doses of insulin will be required
d. Saline will be infused
e. Potassium depletion will have to be corrected

155

This girl is very keen on sports. She spends an hour in the gym, then plays tennis during the morning break. She does not like her school lunch and leaves half of it. Her friends notice that she seems light-headed and confused and she falls asleep in the afternoon lesson. Her hypoglycaemia can be relieved by:

a. An intramuscular injection of adrenaline
b. An injection of glucagon
c. A drink containing sugar
d. 10 units of insulin, intramuscularly
e. 100 mg of hydrocortisone, intramuscularly

153

a. **True** – The diet and insulin dosage must be arranged to produce the optimum levels of blood glucose
b. **True** – How and when to give insulin
c. **True** – Including what steps should be taken to relieve the condition
d. **False** – Intravenous injection not given by a relative
e. **True**

154

a. **False** – It should be given intravenously (or sometimes intramuscularly)
b. **True**
c. **False** – When given by intravenous pump, about 5 units per hour are required, depending on the level of blood glucose
d. **True**
e. **True**

155

a. **False**
b. **True**
c. **True**
d. **False** – Dangerous
e. **False**

156

The following points should be remembered about the administration of insulin:

a. The standard strength of insulin is 100 units per ml
b. Patients should be taught to give themselves insulin intramuscularly
c. The injection site should be cleaned with spirit
d. The action of soluble insulin lasts about 8 hours
e. A bottle of insulin in use may be stored for up to 1 month at room temperature

157

Human, rather than animal, insulin is preferred:

a. When insulin causes a local reaction after injection
b. For patients starting on insulin
c. In elderly patients
d. For patients who develop an allergy to animal insulin
e. For diabetic women who are pregnant

158

The degree of diabetic control can be monitored by:

a. Testing the urine for glucose
b. Estimating the blood cholesterol level
c. Measurement of the blood glucose level by the patient at home
d. Measurement of the glycosylated haemoglobin (HbA) concentration in the blood
e. Estimation of the salivary glucose concentration

159

Which of the following may alter a patient's insulin requirements?

a. Major surgery
b. Pregnancy
c. ACE inhibitors
d. Changing from animal to human insulin
e. Severe intercurrent infection

156

a. **True**
b. **False** – Insulin is given subcutaneously for routine treatment
c. **False** – Spirit hardens the skin
d. **True**
e. **True** – For prolonged storage it should be kept between 4 to 8°C, but not frozen

157

a. **True**
b. **True**
c. **False**
d. **True**
e. **True**

158

a. **True** – But not a very sensitive method
b. **False** – But should be performed in diabetic subjects as they have an extra risk of atheroma
c. **True**
d. **True** – Gives an indication of blood glucose levels over a long period of time
e. **False**

159

a. **True** – Modification of dosage regimen necessary
b. **True** – Change to human insulin
c. **False**
d. **True** – Slightly lower dose of human insulin may be needed
e. **True** – Raised dose of insulin required

160

A 60-year-old overweight housewife has non-insulin-dependent (type II) diabetes. Attempts to control her disorder by diet have failed and she has been prescribed one of the sulphonylurea drugs. You provide the following information:

a. They replace the need for a weight-controlling diet
b. They stimulate the release of insulin from the pancreas
c. They never cause hypoglycaemia
d. They may cause loss of appetite
e. They are given before retiring at night as a single dose

161

An obese middle-aged man surges into the 'Healthy Man' clinic for his appointment. His job leads to a sedentary lifestyle, interspersed with many good dinners. He tells you that it is time he lost some weight. Which of the following are true?

a. He will have to reduce his intake to 750 kcals per day
b. The object of any diet is to reduce body mass index (BMI) to 30
c. Obesity is strongly associated with the development of non-insulin-dependent diabetes
d. He can try taking fenfluramine to reduce his appetite
e. He can try taking thyroxine to stimulate metabolism and reduce weight

162

A young woman comes to the clinic where you work as a family planning nurse to ask if she can take the 'Pill'. You explain that the combined pill, which is most commonly prescribed, operates by:

a. Destroying the male sperm in the vagina
b. Making the endometrium (lining of the uterus) less suitable for implantation
c. Inhibiting ovulation
d. Reducing the motility of the fallopian tubes
e. Altering the cervical mucus, which makes it more difficult for the sperm to penetrate

160

a. **False** – It is important not to gain weight
b. **True**
c. **False**
d. **False**
e. **False** – It is given with breakfast and also during the day

161

a. **True**
b. **False** – The BMI should be 20–25
c. **True**
d. **True** – But it is only of limited value and should not be used for more than 3 months
e. **False** – Thyroxine may be dangerous if used for this purpose

162

a. **False**
b. **True**
c. **True**
d. **False**
e. **True**

163

You take a careful nursing history from her to ensure that she has none of the following disorders which would contraindicate taking the combined pill:

a. Asthma
b. A history of thrombo-embolic disease
c. Severe hypertension
d. Tuberculosis
e. Carcinoma of the breast

164

She needs to be aware of possible side-effects of the combined pill. These include:

a. Nausea
b. Venous thrombosis
c. Hypertension
d. Ovarian carcinoma
e. Vascular disease

165

She also needs instruction in taking the combined contraceptive pill:

a. The course should be started on the fourth day of her menstrual cycle
b. The combined pill should be taken daily, before retiring for the night
c. If the combined pill is taken more than 12 hours late, protection may be lost
d. The combined pill should be stopped 4 weeks before elective surgery
e. Before taking a new drug, ensure that it does not reduce the efficacy of the contraceptive

163

a. **False**
b. **True**
c. **True**
d. **False** — But remember that rifampicin, which is given to treat tuberculosis, reduces the efficacy of the 'Pill' by increasing estrogen elimination
e. **True**

164

a. **True**
b. **True** — Due to estrogen content
c. **True**
d. **False**
e. **True** — Due to progestogen content, but adverse effects in a healthy, non-smoking young woman are few compared with the problems associated with an unwanted pregnancy

165

a. **False** — Start on the first day of the cycle: on the fourth day or after, protection may be lost
b. **False** — It is taken at approximately the same time each day: the actual time does not matter
c. **True**
d. **True**
e. **True**

166

Which of the following would indicate that she should stop taking the combined pill and seek immediate medical advice?

a. Pain across the chest
b. Coughing up blood/shortness of breath
c. Nausea
d. Pain and swelling in her calf
e. Severe headache with visual disturbance

167

An 18-year-old student arrives at the clinic in a panic. Last night she had unprotected intercourse and fears she will become pregnant. You tell her:

a. She runs an up to 20% risk of pregnancy, depending on the stage of her menstrual cycle
b. Pregnancy can be prevented by taking a low estrogen pill within 48 hours
c. It can also be prevented by taking an aperient
d. The best prevention is by taking two doses of a high estrogen pill within 3 days of exposure
e. Inserting an IUD is the only method of preventing pregnancy after 72 hours

168

A 50-year-old business executive is considering hormone replacement therapy (HRT), but has heard a number of unfavourable reports relating to its safety. You are able to reassure her of its positive effects on health:

a. It reduces the risk of osteoporosis
b. It decreases the risk of cardiovascular disease
c. It decreases the risk of breast cancer
d. It can be administered as a patch applied to the skin
e. Some preparations avoid the problem of monthly bleeding

166

a. **True** – Possible coronary thrombosis
b. **True** – Possible pulmonary embolus
c. **False** – Not an emergency, although it can be a side-effect
d. **True** – Possible venous thrombosis
e. **True** – Possible cerebral vascular disturbance

167

a. **True**
b. **False**
c. **False**
d. **True**
e. **True**

168

a. **True**
b. **True**
c. **False** – There is a slightly increased risk, especially after five years of HRT
d. **True**
e. **True**

169

A 28-year-old housewife suffers from appalling premenstrual tension. Last month she cried for 3 days and is worried about her relationship with her family, especially her husband, who is not considerate. Which of the following may help?

a. Thyroxine
b. The combined oral contraceptive Pill
c. Gamolenic acid (evening primrose oil)
d. Fluoxetine, a 5HT re-uptake inhibitor antidepressant
e. Thiazide diuretics

170

Which of these drugs may be used after delivery to cause the uterus to contract?

a. Ritodrine
b. Ergometrine
c. An NSAIA
d. Oxytocin
e. Carboprost

171

Prostaglandins are widespread throughout the body and have a variety of actions:

a. They cause the redness, swelling and pain of inflammation
b. Their actions are increased by NSAIAs
c. They are involved in thrombosis
d. They have a protective action on the gastric mucosa
e. They relax uterine muscle

169

a. **False**
b. **True** – Suppresses the menstrual cycle
c. **True**
d. **True**
e. **True** – Often used, but rarely helps. It is a difficult disorder to relieve and often many treatments are tried

170

a. **False** – Inhibits uterine contraction
b. **True**
c. **False** – Inhibits uterine contraction
d. **True**
e. **True**

171

a. **True**
b. **False** – Actions decreased by NSAIAs
c. **True**
d. **True**
e. **False** – They cause contractions

Drugs affecting renal function

Diuretics are widely prescribed to relieve salt and water retention and to treat hypertension. Patients usually need to take these drugs over long periods, often with minimal supervision. Their side-effects can be annoying, especially to elderly people, who are the group most often requiring them. Good patient education is essential to ensure that diuretics are taken as prescribed and that side-effects are avoided.

172

A 60-year-old retired man is suffering from cardiac failure. The thiazide diuretics that have been prescribed for him may cause which of the following?

a. Gout
b. Lung fibrosis
c. Hypercalcaemia
d. Potassium depletion leading to digitalis toxicity
e. Decreased glucose tolerance

173

Loop diuretics (e.g. frusemide) have certain advantages over thiazide diuretics:

a. They act more quickly
b. They are more powerful
c. They are particularly effective in the treatment of hypertension
d. They do not cause potassium depletion
e. They can be given intravenously

174

A patient is suffering from potassium depletion as a result of treatment with a thiazide diuretic. The thiazide is replaced by a potassium-sparing diuretic (amiloride). You are asked to check that this will not interact with other drugs he is taking. These include:

a. Salbutamol
b. An ACE inhibitor
c. Supplementary potassium
d. Diazepam
e. Sennokot

172

a. **True** – Due to uric acid retention
b. **False**
c. **False** – Although there is decreased calcium excretion by the kidneys
d. **True**
e. **True** – With prolonged treatment

173

a. **True**
b. **True**
c. **False**
d. **False**
e. **True** – There are, at present, no thiazide preparations for intravenous use

174

a. **False**
b. **True** – Potassium retention can occur
c. **True** – Retention can also occur
d. **False**
e. **False**

Chemotherapeutic agents and antibiotics

Antibiotics have revolutionized the treatment of infection so that many previously fatal diseases can now be treated successfully. However, many bacteria have become resistant to antibiotics and the search for new drugs and modifications to older ones continues. Infection remains common, especially among the very young and very old, and approximately 10% of hospital patients develop nosocomial (not present or incubating before admission) infection. Nurses in hospital or the community spend much time preparing and administering antibiotics and they have a vital role in educating patients to take them correctly and appreciate that inappropriate use can contribute to bacterial resistance.

175

A 24-year-old woman is admitted to hospital with meningococcal meningitis. She is treated with large doses of benzylpenicillin. This antibiotic was chosen because:

a. The infecting organism is sensitive to it
b. Benzylpenicillin penetrates easily into the cerebrospinal fluid
c. It can be given in large doses without toxic effects
d. Benzylpenicillin is cheap
e. It can be given by injection

176

An elderly woman, not in the best of health, has had major abdominal surgery. Three days after operation, she says her wound feels sore and the swab you take reveals infection with a staphylococcus, resistant to benzylpenicillin. Which of the following antibiotics could be used to treat her infection?

a. Vancomycin
b. Flucloxacillin
c. Amoxycillin
d. Tetracycline
e. Sodium fusidate

177

A 16-year-old boy develops a sore throat and fever, which are treated with ampicillin. A week later, after responding poorly, he develops a rash. Which of the following are true?

a. Many sore throats are due to viruses
b. Some are due to *Streptococcus pyogenes*
c. Ampicillin is not always the correct antibiotic for a sore throat
d. The rash may be caused by ampicillin
e. His elder sister has cystitis and treats herself with his capsules. Are they likely to be effective?

175

a. **True** – It is essential to choose the correct antibiotic for a given infection
b. **False** – Benzylpenicillin penetrates rather poorly into the cerebrospinal fluid, therefore a large dose is required. In general, an antibiotic must reach the site of infection
c. **True** – Toxicity is important in the choice of antibiotic
d. **True**
e. **True** – A rapid therapeutic effect is thus obtained

176

a. **True** – It is rather toxic, but is effective against methicillin-resistant *Staphylococci* (MRSA), which are resistant to all other antibiotics. It is therefore reserved for MRSA infections
b. **True** – Provided the organism is not resistant
c. **False**
d. **False**
e. **True** – Though resistance may emerge and it should be combined with another antibiotic against staphylococci

177

a. **True** – Therefore do not respond to antibiotics
b. **True**
c. **True** – Correct for a streptococcal infection, but useless for a viral infection
d. **True** – Ampicillin can cause a rash, particularly if the sore throat is due to glandular fever
e. **True** – Cystitis is usually due to *Escherichia coli*, which is usually sensitive to ampicillin, but it is a very bad principle to use other people's drugs

178

Although cephalosporins have a wide spectrum of antibacterial action, they are rarely the first choice in treating infection because:

a. They contain a β lactam ring
b. Most cephalosporins can only be given by injection
c. Most are expensive
d. They can induce allergic responses in those patients who are sensitive to penicillin
e. They taste disgusting so patients do not comply well with treatment

179

As a nurse working with acutely ill patients in an intensive care unit, you are aware that gentamicin (an aminoglycoside):

a. Can be given by mouth to achieve a systemic effect
b. Requires caution in use because it is ototoxic and nephrotoxic
c. Has a narrow therapeutic range, so dosage must be closely monitored
d. Crosses the blood–brain barrier readily
e. Its elimination is not affected by changes in renal function

180

A vagrant has developed pulmonary tuberculosis. He complains that he has to take too many different tablets and wants to know whether the number can be reduced. You explain that several antibiotics have to be taken at the same time to:

a. Prevent the bacteria developing resistance to the antibiotics
b. Eradicate the infection completely
c. Build up his immunity
d. Reduce toxicity
e. Improve compliance

178

a. **True** – And therefore have many similar properties to penicillin
b. **True**
c. **True**
d. **True**
e. **False**

179

a. **False** – By injection
b. **True**
c. **True** – Blood level should be taken before and 1 hour after dosing
d. **False**
e. **False**

180

a. **True**
b. **True**
c. **False**
d. **False**
e. **False** – Good compliance is essential, but complicated regimens contribute to poor compliance

181

The following drugs are commonly used in treating tuberculosis:

a. Vancomycin
b. Isoniazid
c. Rifampicin
d. Clindamycin
e. Pyrazinamide

182

Which of these items of information should be given to young patients who are treated with rifampicin?

a. It must be taken as a single dose, before breakfast, each day
b. It can cause jaundice with nausea and vomiting
c. It will stain tears and urine pink
d. It will reduce the efficacy of oral contraceptives
e. It will make them feel drowsy, so they should not drive

183

The quinolone antibiotic ciprofloxacin is used to treat several types of infection likely to be seen by nurses, but it has a number of potential side-effects:

a. It can induce fits in epileptic patients
b. It can cause photosensitivity
c. It can enhance the effects of alcohol
d. It is deposited as crystals in the urine, unless taken with at least 3 litres of fluid daily
e. It may damage weight-bearing joints in children

181

a. **False**
b. **True**
c. **True**
d. **False**
e. **True**

Rifampicin, Isoniazid and Pyrazinamide are frequently used in combination.

182

a. **True**
b. **True** — And also transient disturbances of liver function tests
c. **True**
d. **True**
e. **False**

183

a. **True**
b. **True** — Avoid sunlight
c. **True**
d. **True**
e. **True** — Also stop if symptoms of tendon inflammation develop

184

As a practice nurse you often have to advise patients about taking antibiotics. Which of the following information should they receive?

a. They should take the full course, even if the infection appears to have resolved before the antibiotics are finished
b. They should take the full course, even if they show signs of allergy to the drug
c. They may experience mild diarrhoea
d. Loss of concentration is a little-discussed side-effect of taking antibiotics
e. They should report any previous allergies or adverse effects from drugs to the doctor before starting treatment

185

A 50-year-old woman has developed candidiasis and clotrimazole pessaries and cream have been prescribed for her. She will need the following information:

a. The pessaries must be inserted three times a day
b. The pessaries must be inserted every night before retiring
c. She should destroy all her underwear as it will be highly contagious
d. Her urine will be tested for glucose
e. Her partner (if any) should also be treated with clotrimazole cream

186

In the prevention of post-operative infection:

a. Antibiotics should be started 48 hours before operation
b. If gentamicin and penicillin are used together, they should not be mixed in the same infusion bottle
c. Antibiotics should not be given as a bolus into the infusion line
d. It is usually necessary to continue the antibiotic for at least a week post-operatively
e. If metronidazole is used, alcohol must be avoided

184

a. **True**
b. **False** — Consult the doctor
c. **True** — Diarrhoea is fairly common, but, if severe, should be taken seriously as it may indicate bowel infection with a resistant organism
d. **False** — But ciprofloxacin enhances the effect of alcohol and may interfere with driving
e. **True** — Very important

185

a. **False** — 200 mg for three nights or 500 mg for one night
b. **True**
c. **False**
d. **True** — May complicate diabetes
e. **True**

186

a. **False** — Two hours is optimum
b. **True**
c. **False**
d. **False** — Usually up to 24 hours post-operatively
e. **True** — Together they cause a toxic reaction

187

Accidental viral infection is an occupational risk for nurses:

a. Active immunization is available against hepatitis A and B, but not hepatitis C at present
b. HIV infection can occur through the intact skin
c. The possibility of HIV infection occurring from a needle-stick injury with infected blood is about 1 : 500
d. Treatment with zidovudine will prevent infection
e. Contamination with HIV infected body fluids can effectively be treated with 1% hypochlorite solution

187

a. **True**
b. **False** – but gloves should be worn and hands washed when handling any blood/body fluids
c. **True**
d. **False**
e. **True**

Sera, vaccines and antihistamines

The human body is continually subjected to the risk of infection by micro-organisms or to damage by toxins produced by bacteria. Fortunately, natural immunity can be enhanced by immunization. This procedure is commonly performed by health visitors, school nurses and practice nurses. Anyone responsible for administering immunization should be aware of contraindications, the special precautions which should be taken with live vaccines, how to recognize adverse reactions and the action to take. Such nurses also play a key part in making the public aware of the benefits conferred by immunization, dispelling myths, encouraging uptake and maintaining records. Some disorders are due to an overactive immune system, so drugs have been introduced which suppress immunity, or some aspect of the immune reaction. The more powerful of these drugs are two-edged as they may leave the body's defences open to infection. In the management of these patients, careful observation and monitoring are essential.

188

Before a teaching session on the use of vaccines, you need to ensure that your students/colleagues have an adequate understanding of the immune system. Which of the following are true?

a. Antigens activate the immune system
b. In humoral immunity, the immune system is stimulated to produce antibodies
c. In cell-mediated immunity, the immune system produces sensitized lymphocytes
d. Immunoglobulins obtained from human serum are safer than those derived from animals
e. T-Cells are important in cell-mediated immunity

189

For an immunization programme in a general practice, the following should be available because of the rare possibility of an anaphylactic reaction:

a. Morphine for injection
b. Chlorpheniramine (an antihistamine) for injection
c. Adrenaline 1 : 1000 solution
d. Oxygen
e. Hydrocortisone for injection

190

As a nurse employed in a residential home, you recommend the following vaccinations for elderly diabetic people:

a. Hib immunization against *Haemophilus influenzae*
b. Influenza vaccine
c. Rubella vaccine
d. Pneumococcal vaccine
e. Staphylococcal vaccine

188

a. **True** – May be bacteria, toxins or other substances
b. **True**
c. **True**
d. **True** – Less chance of an allergic reaction
e. **True**

189

a. **False**
b. **True**
c. **True**
d. **True**
e. **True**

190

a. **False** – Usually used in young children
b. **True**
c. **False** – Not necessary in that age group
d. **True**
e. **False** – Not available

191

As a health visitor, you invite parents to bring infants less than 12 months old to receive the following:

a. Triple vaccine (Diphtheria, Tetanus, Pertussis)
b. BCG vaccine
c. Polio vaccine
d. Hib vaccine
e. Rubella vaccine

192

There are several contraindications to immunization with live vaccines. They include:

a. A severe general reaction to the last dose of vaccine
b. Immunization of an HIV positive subject with polio vaccine
c. Patients taking large doses of corticosteroids
d. A family history of convulsions
e. Patients with leukaemia

193

A young man has troublesome hayfever and asthma and seeks your advice about antihistamines. You tell him:

a. All antihistamines are sedating
b. They will not help to improve his asthma
c. Some antihistamines have anti-emetic properties
d. He will need a doctor's prescription to obtain antihistamines
e. Antihistamine ointment should be applied locally to bites or stings

194

Drugs which suppress the immune system can be used to:

a. Suppress antibody production
b. Treat osteoarthritis
c. Prevent rejection of transplanted organs
d. Boost the neutrophil count
e. Reduce inflammatory responses (e.g. in rheumatoid arthritis)

191

a. **True**
b. **False** – 10–14 years, earlier if in close contact with open tuberculosis
c. **True**
d. **True**
e. **False** – 2 years with MMR or later in childhood

192

a. **True**
b. **False** – Contraindications to vaccines in HIV positive subjects: see *Immunisation Against Infectious Diseases*, HMSO
c. **True**
d. **False**
e. **True**

193

a. **False** – Several (e.g. terfenadine) are non-sedating
b. **True**
c. **True** – e.g. promethazine
d. **False** – Some are available 'over the counter' (e.g. astemizole, terfenadine)
e. **False** – Risk of hypersensitivity, therefore best avoided

194

a. **True**
b. **False**
c. **True** – Cyclosporin is used to reduce cellular immunity
d. **False** – Some will lower the white cell count
e. **True**

Drugs used to treat tropical diseases

Tropical diseases, like their background, are inclined to be dramatic and florid. The majority are infective and can be treated with drugs. The problem of dealing with them is no longer lack of knowledge but of providing effective care in the primitive conditions which prevail in many parts of the tropics. Knowledge about tropical diseases and their treatment is not confined to health professionals aspiring to voluntary work overseas: air travel has brought tropical diseases much nearer home for it is possible to catch malaria in Central Africa but not be taken ill until after arrival in London. Some knowledge of tropical diseases is thus worth cultivating for any member of the nursing profession.

195

Malaria prophylaxis is essential when visiting many parts of the world, but the drugs have a number of side-effects:

a. Proguanil – jaundice
b. Quinine – headaches and tinnitus
c. Mefloquine – hallucination and mental upsets
d. Chloroquine – arthritis
e. Primaquine – haemolysis of red cells in certain sensitive subjects

196

A woman is embarking on a cruise around the world and will leave the ship for a few nights to travel inland to some regions where malaria remains a problem. You give her the following information:

a. Prophylactic drugs should be started on arrival in the malarious area
b. The use of mosquito nets is unnecessary
c. The prophylaxis required varies in different parts of the world
d. Treatment should be continued for 1 week after leaving the malarious area
e. Up to date advice can be obtained from the Malaria Reference Laboratory

197

Pierre Lapin, aged 7, has a threadworm infestation. His health visitor is likely to recommend:

a. A single dose of mebendazole
b. Camomile tea
c. An aperient
d. Treating the whole family
e. Scrubbing fingernails before meals

195

a. **False**
b. **True**
c. **True**
d. **False**
e. **True** – Those with an inherited abnormality of the red blood cells

196

a. **False** – 1 week before arrival (2 weeks for mefloquine)
b. **False**
c. **True** – Due to resistant strains
d. **False** – 1 month
e. **True**

197

a. **True**
b. **False**
c. **False** – Not necessary
d. **True**
e. **True**

Vitamins and drugs used to treat anaemia

Deficiency of a particular vitamin will lead to a specific disease, but providing that a good mixed diet is taken, there is no advantage to be gained from extra doses of vitamins in healthy subjects. However, some people may have a poorly balanced diet or be unable, because of disease, to absorb or use vitamins so deficiencies can still occur.

Anaemia is usually caused by a deficiency of iron which, in turn, may be due to a poor diet, failure of absorption or chronic blood loss. Other types of anaemia are due to a lack of certain essential factors or to damage to the bone marrow.

Discussion about diet and deficiencies is popular nowadays and many claims are made for a wide range of dietary elements. Nurses need to be aware of what is really important in the diet and to realize that excess may be as harmful as deficiency.

198

Vitamins are a popular subject for discussion and you may be asked about them. Which is true?

a. Vitamin D can be dangerous if the correct dose is exceeded
b. High doses of vitamin C prevent cancer
c. Vitamin E prevents coronary artery disease
d. Eating fish regularly reduces the risk of coronary artery disease
e. High doses of vitamin B_1 improve the intelligence of normal adults

199

Which of these diseases can be caused by a vitamin deficiency?

a. Osteomalacia
b. Pernicious anaemia
c. Duodenal ulcer
d. Beri-beri
e. Haemolytic anaemia

200

The following diseases can lead to a related vitamin deficiency:

a. Alcoholism
b. Chronic renal failure
c. Diabetes
d. Malabsorption syndrome
e. Epilepsy

201

Iron deficiency may cause:

a. Numbness of hands and feet
b. Microcytic anaemia
c. A smooth tongue
d. Muscle wasting
e. Undue fatigue

198

a. **True** – Increases the amount of calcium in the blood
b. **False** – No good evidence
c. **True** – Probably
d. **True**
e. **False**

199

a. **True** – Vitamin D deficiency
b. **True** – Vitamin B_{12} (cyanocobalamin) deficiency
c. **False**
d. **True** – Vitamin B_1 deficiency
e. **False**

200

a. **True** – Vitamin B_1
b. **True** – Vitamin D resistance develops
c. **False**
d. **True** – Multivitamin deficiency
e. **False** – But phenytoin can increase the breakdown of vitamin D

201

a. **False**
b. **True**
c. **True**
d. **False**
e. **True**

202

A woman who has been eating poorly and also suffers from heavy periods has developed iron-deficiency anaemia. Her GP tells her she will need drugs, but her husband has heard rumours about iron preparations and wants answers to specific questions. Which of the following ideas are true?

a. She will need to take drugs by mouth for 4 months after her haemoglobin has been restored to normal
b. Intramuscular injections may stain the skin unless a specific technique is used in administration
c. She must store her tablets in a safe place as overdose can be fatal
d. Iron can also be used to cure pernicious anaemia
e. She will need to take folic acid tablets

203

Which of the following supplements will be prescribed for a pregnant woman?

a. Vitamin A
b. Folic acid
c. Hydroxocobalamin
d. Iron
e. Vitamin E

202

a. **True** – To replace iron stores
b. **True**
c. **True**
d. **False** – Hydroxocobalamin is required
e. **False** – Unless folate-deficent as well; or she is pregnant

203

a. **False** – Excess may cause birth defects, so only given in special circumstances
b. **True** – Deficiency may develop and it also reduces the chance of neural tube defects
c. **False**
d. **True**
e. **False**

Drugs used to treat malignant disease

The use of cytotoxic drugs in the treatment of patients with malignant disease demands a high level of expertise on the part of the nurse. Increasingly, patients receive care through specialist oncology services. Nurses employed as part of the multidisciplinary team will have taken additional qualifications which allow them to develop expertise in the administration of cytotoxic chemotherapy, to monitor the patient for response to treatment, to be alert for side-effects and to know how to alleviate or minimize them. Today patients tend to be treated as outpatients or may even have their drugs administered by a nurse visiting their home. They are likely to face many of the disagreeable effects of chemotherapy without the immediate support of a health professional and must therefore be prepared by the nurse to recognize adverse effects and to initiate the appropriate self-care action. Ability to communicate with outpatients, to educate them about their drugs and to tolerate their side-effects are of paramount importance. Lack of understanding and poor symptom control frequently result in the refusal of further potentially curative treatment.

204

Cytotoxic drugs can be used in various ways to achieve different objectives. Which of the following is true?

a. Combination chemotherapy (using more than one drug at a time) is often more effective than a single drug
b. The aim of chemotherapy may not necessarily be cure
c. Adjuvant therapy is necessary for all patients after an operation to remove the cancer
d. Not all types of malignancy respond to chemotherapy
e. Cancer chemotherapy is best when carried out in a specialized unit

205

Which of the following drugs cause severe tissue damage if extravasation occurs at the infusion site?

a. Bleomycin
b. Vincristine
c. Doxorubicin
d. Ifosphamide
e. Mustine (chlormethine)

206

Which normal tissues are especially liable to be damaged by cytotoxic drugs?

a. Brain
b. Intestinal mucosa
c. Muscle
d. Bone marrow
e. Adzenals

204

a. **True**
b. **True** – Palliation is sometimes very effective
c. **False** – It depends on the type of cancer and other factors
d. **True**
e. **True**

205

a. **False**
b. **True**
c. **True**
d. **False**
e. **True**

206

a. **False**
b. **True** – Both oral and gut
c. **False**
d. **True** – Usually white cells or platelets affected
e. **False**

207

Which of the following cytotoxic drugs are markedly emetic?

a. Doxorubicin (adriamycin)
b. Vincristine
c. Bleomycin
d. Cisplatin
e. High-dose cyclophosphamide

208

Which of these malignancies can often be *cured* by cytotoxic drugs?

a. Testicular cancer
b. Acute lymphoblastic leukaemia in children
c. Carcinoma of the bronchus
d. Hodgkin's disease
e. Melanoma

209

A patient with a lymphoma attends the oncology clinic at regular intervals for combination drug treatment which includes doxorubicin (adriamycin). Which of the following apply?

a. The injection of doxorubicin should be given into the brachial vein
b. A No. 23 butterfly needle or cannula can be used
c. An anti-emetic should be given 1 hour after the injection
d. If extravasation occurs the infusion should be slowed
e. The occurrence of extravasation should be reported to a doctor

207

a. **True**
b. **False**
c. **False**
d. **True**
e. **True**

208

a. **True**
b. **True**
c. **False**
d. **True**
e. **False**

209

Doxorubicin is a very irritant drug, as are several other cytotoxic drugs, so if these drugs are given intravenously, great care is needed to avoid tissue damage and preserve veins for future use

a. **False** – If the brachial vein is damaged, venous access to the arm can be compromised
b. **True** – Cannula preferred for irritant drugs
c. **False** – Anti-emetics should be given before treatment to prevent vomiting as this is easier than relieving it
d. **False** – Stop the infusion and try to withdraw some of the drug. Oncology units will have their own guidelines to deal with extravasation
e. **True** – It can cause an area of serious necrosis

210

A woman is being treated with cytotoxic drugs as an outpatient. Which of the following requires *urgent* referral to the oncology unit?

a. Bruising
b. High fever
c. Hair loss
d. Jaundice
e. Severe necrotic reaction at the injection site

211

As many patients with certain types of cancer are now cured, they should be told the possible long-term risks of treatment, which include:

a. Permanent sterility in men is possible
b. Fetal abnormality if the patient is pregnant during treatment
c. Women cannot become pregnant after treatment
d. A secondary malignancy may develop after treatment
e. Hair loss, which occurs with some drugs, is permanent

212

Which of these hormones or hormone antagonists are used in treating malignant disease?

a. Oxytocin
b. Stilboestrol (diethylstilbestrol)
c. Tamoxifen
d. Corticosteroids
e. Goserelin

210

a. **True** – May be due to platelet deficiency
b. **True** – Probably infection associated with low white blood cell count
c. **False** – Not an emergency
d. **True** – Suggests liver damage
e. **True**

Patients receiving cancer chemotherapy require careful and well organized supervision

211

a. **True** – But this is not inevitable and depends on the drugs used
b. **True** – Women should wait 6 months after finishing treatment before trying to conceive. There may also be prognostic, social and financial problems to be considered
c. **False**
d. **True** – The chance of this happening depends on the drugs used and whether there is additional radiotherapy
e. **False** – The hair regrows after treatment finishes

212

a. **False**
b. **True** – Carcinoma of the prostate
c. **True** – Carcinoma of the breast
d. **True** – Lymphomas and some leukaemias
e. **True** – Carcinoma of the prostate

Certain cancers (e.g. breast and prostate) are hormone-dependent. Drugs which block the action of the relevant hormone suppress the cancer; however, although it is possible to produce a remission, this form of treatment is not curative

Drugs during pregnancy and in old age

Members of the public are keenly aware of the dangers of taking drugs throughout pregnancy and may ask health professionals about the risks associated with medication, including over the counter drugs. The problem is more difficult if the woman is taking drugs for an established disorder, or when drugs have been taken in the early weeks before pregnancy was suspected. Increasingly women and their partners are invited by midwives and health visitors for preconceptual counselling, so they can be made aware of the risks of drugs at this time. Also, changes can be made to any prescriptions the woman may need for existing disorders.

Elderly people make up a high proportion of patients admitted to hospital, account for many visits by nurses in the community and for numerous consultations with practice nurses. Particular problems are associated with drug treatment in the elderly patients and many stem from the prescription of several drugs to tackle a range of disorders in one individual. For patients at home, this can lead to confusion and mistakes. It has been estimated that drug-related problems are responsible for 10–30% of admissions of elderly patients to hospital. Once in hospital, it is likely that the former drug regimen will be adjusted and the patient will need time to learn the new regimen well before discharge.

The ageing process is accompanied by a number of physiological changes which may affect the metabolism and excretion of many drugs: this has practical implications for the administration, timing of dosage and monitoring of response and adverse effects. All nurses need to be fully conversant with both the physiological and psycho-social effects of drug treatment in these patients.

213

The use of drugs in pregnancy may carry risks. Which of the following are true?

a. Few drugs cross the placenta and reach the fetus
b. The fetus is most at risk from drug damage during the first 3 months of pregnancy
c. About 2% of babies have some abnormality at birth, even if no drugs are taken
d. 50% of abnormalities are due to drugs
e. In the UK, at least 80% of women take some drug during pregnancy

214

The following 'over the counter drugs' can be used safely during pregnancy provided that the correct dose is not exceeded:

a. Promethazine
b. Astemizole
c. Cimetidine
d. Ibuprofen
e. Aspirin

215

A woman who is 2 months pregnant is taking a holiday in a remote part of the world. She has listed the drugs she thinks would be completely safe for her to use if she were ill. These include:

a. Paracetamol
b. Amoxycillin
c. Quinine
d. Phenytoin
e. Diazepam

213

a. **False** – Most drugs cross the placental barrier
b. **True**
c. **True** – This is important when considering the problem of whether a particular drug causes fetal abnormalities
d. **False** – About 5% are drug-related
e. **False** – About 30%

214

a. **True** – But not in the last 2 weeks of pregnancy due to excitability of the neonate
b. **False** – Evidence of toxicity
c. **True** ⎱ Both these drugs carry little, if any, risk, but caution
d. **True** ⎰ is advised
e. **False** – There can be problems in late pregnancy: increased length of labour and blood loss; neonatal jaundice

It is very difficult to say a drug is *completely* safe, so many drugs carry a warning. Risks must be balanced against benefit.

215

a. **True**
b. **True**
c. **False** – Quinine can be teratogenic, but the risk of malaria is greater
d. **False** – Phenytoin can cause fetal abnormalities, but fits are also dangerous
e. **True** – But at birth the neonate's respiration can be depressed

Appendix 4 in the *British National Formulary* lists the dangers of drugs in pregnancy

216

The correct dose of a drug for a child may differ from that for an adult because:

a. Bioavailability differs considerably
b. There are differences in body composition
c. There are differences in body weight
d. There are possible differences in elimination
e. There are differences in body temperature

217

Adverse reactions to drugs occur more frequently in elderly patients. This may be because:

a. They take more drugs
b. They take less exercise
c. Their compliance may be poor and muddled
d. Elimination may be reduced
e. They often have a poor diet

218

Which of these drugs require reduced dosage in elderly patients?

a. Amoxycillin
b. Gentamicin
c. Tricyclic antidepressants
d. Digoxin
e. Paracetamol

219

Are these drugs especially appropriate in elderly patients?

a. Thioridazine – for restlessness with paranoia at night
b. Anticholinergics – for Parkinson's disease
c. Tolbutamide – for non-insulin-dependent diabetes
d. Cimetidine – for peptic ulcers
e. Thiazide diuretics – for hypertension

216

a. **False**
b. **True**
c. **True**
d. **True** – Renal elimination is low in newborn infants, but increases rapidly in the first months of life
e. **False**

217

a. **True**
b. **False**
c. **True** – Leading to overdose
d. **True** – Renal function declines with age and leads to higher blood levels of drugs which are excreted by the kidneys
e. **False**

218

a. **False**
b. **True** – Renal excretion may be reduced
c. **True** – They can cause hypotension with fainting, particularly in older people, and, rarely, confusion and fits
d. **True** – Renal excretion is reduced
e. **False**

In general, the dose of all drugs should be kept as low as possible in elderly patients

219

a. **True**
b. **False** – Troublesome side-effects (e.g. urinary retention, glaucoma)
c. **True** – Short-acting, thus less risk of hypoglycaemia
d. **False** – Confusion can occur, but is rare
e. **True** – Easy to use, minimum side-effects, but they may exacerbate diabetes and precipitate gout. However, other hypotensive drugs can be used

Adverse reactions to drugs and testing of drugs

If you have worked through each section of this book in sequence, or even if you have selected particular sections to test specific areas of knowledge, you will be aware that treatment with drugs can be complicated by problems of drug interactions or the adverse reactions associated with individual drugs. These problems are particularly common among elderly patients and those with chronic disorders, who make up a high proportion of the population seen by nurses. This is because such patients often have a combination of health problems and are more likely to be prescribed a cocktail of drugs or have been taking drugs for a long time. Whether in hospital or in the community, the nurse is frequently the health professional with whom the patient has the greatest and most sustained contact. The nurse is therefore in an ideal position to observe side-effects and adverse reactions and is often the patient's first choice when they encounter problems with their drugs. In some instances side-effects may be commonplace and the patient will need only reassurance or advice about some straightforward self-care action, but in others it may be necessary to stop the drug, find a substitute, alter the dose or explore the timing of dosages. Much of the morbidity and mortality associated with drugs comes with those most commonly prescribed. Thus nurses today cannot afford to abdicate their responsibility in dealing with the problems of drug treatment.

220

Adverse reactions to drugs may be due to:

a. Increased sensitivity to the action of the drug
b. Decreased elimination
c. An allergic reaction
d. Genetic factors
e. Unknown factors

221

The danger of adverse reactions to drugs can be minimized by:

a. Reducing drug treatment to a reasonable minimum
b. Only using short-acting drugs
c. Taking a comprehensive drug history
d. Giving drugs by injection if possible
e. Keeping the course of treatment as short as possible

222

Taking a comprehensive drug history is an important part of nurses' duties because:

a. The patient may have had an adverse reaction to a certain drug which should therefore be avoided
b. Some diseases may be drug-induced
c. The patient may already be receiving other drugs so there is a risk of interaction
d. It may be important not to stop certain drugs (e.g. corticosteroids)
e. The previous response of a patient to drugs may be a good guide to further treatment

223

Important interactions occur between these groups of drugs:

a. Oral contraceptives and benzylpenicillin
b. Lithium and thiazide diuretics
c. ACE inhibitors and potassium-sparing diuretics
d. Aminophylline and corticosteroids
e. Monoamine oxidase inhibitors and pethidine

220

a. **True** – Sedatives depress respiration in an asthmatic attack
b. **True** – Usually presenting as too large a dose
c. **True** – Requires previous exposure to the drug
d. **True** – There are various genetic factors involved
e. **True**

221

a. **True**
b. **False**
c. **True** – See next question
d. **False**
e. **True**

The less exposure to drugs, the less chance of an adverse reaction

222

a. **True**
b. **True** – As may changes in the patient's condition
c. **True**
d. **True**
e. **True**

223

a. **False** – But ampicillin and other broad spectrum antibiotics and rifampicin reduce the efficacy of the combined contraceptive pill
b. **True** – Leads to lithium retention
c. **True** – Leads to potassium retention
d. **False**
e. **True** – Central nervous system effects, hyper/hypotension

224

A patient being discharged from hospital is to continue drug treatment at home. He should be told to avoid alcohol as his drug will interact with it. His drug could be:

a. Thiazide diuretics
b. Glyceryl trinitrate
c. Metronidazole
d. Warfarin
e. Griseofulvin

225

You are assisting in the trial of a new drug for depression. In designing the trial it is important:

a. To compare the effect of the drug with a placebo or with a drug already established in treatment
b. To ensure that the populations of patients being treated are similar
c. To include enough patients to make the results meaningful
d. For those carrying out the trial to know whether the subject is taking the new drug or the placebo/established drug
e. To decide on clear objectives and criteria before starting the trial

226

Which of these statements are correct?

a. A placebo is a substance which has no pharmacological effect, but may produce a therapeutic effect
b. Generic prescribing means prescribing only those drugs which are in the *British National Formulary*
c. Ethics committees are set up to ensure that patients are given the correct treatment
d. Many hospitals have their own formularies which usually list the drugs kept in the pharmacy and considered most appropriate for use
e. The 'yellow card' is a warning card given to doctors whose prescribing record is poor

224

a. **False**
b. **False**
c. **True** – Nausea, flushing
d. **True** – Effect enhanced
e. **True** – Headache, flushing

225

a. **True**
b. **True** – There are different types of depression which may vary in their response to a drug – like must be compared with like
c. **True** – This is a matter of statistical analysis and requires estimation of the probability that the result is significant and not due to chance
d. **False** – Observer bias may produce misleading results if the observer knows which is being used. Most trials are carried out 'double blind'
e. **True** – If this is not done the result of the trial may be muddled or even meaningless

226

a. **True**
b. **False** – Generic prescribing means prescribing a drug by its approved name rather than its brand name
c. **False** – They grant approval for research on patients or normal volunteers
d. **True**
e. **False** – Doctors and dentists should report adverse effects of drugs to the Committee for the Safety of Medicines on a specially prepared 'yellow card' which is widely available

Drug dependence (drug addiction)

Nurses employed in a range of settings will encounter patients who have become drug dependent: in the A&E department, dealing with acute withdrawal symptoms and providing care for people who are experiencing the physical and psycho-social effects of drug dependence. The knowledge that drug dependence and substance abuse are common within the general population also has profound implications for the safe custody of drugs everywhere.

227

Which of these factors contribute to drug dependence?

a. Availability of drugs
b. Cultural and social factors
c. Individual personality
d. Poverty
e. Possible biochemical susceptibility

228

A 26-year-old patient attends the A&E department claiming to be an opioid addict and to be suffering withdrawal symptoms. What steps should be taken?

a. Look for evidence of drug abuse and for withdrawal signs
b. Treat withdrawal symptoms symptomatically
c. If requiring admission, give a small dose of diamorphine (heroin) by mouth
d. Give 10 ml of methadone mixture (10 mg) by mouth if symptoms are severe
e. Maintenance should be started with 100 mg of methadone daily

229

Nurses and others should not smoke because it increases the risk of:

a. Vascular disease
b. Migraine
c. Cancer of the lung and lip
d. Diabetes
e. Thrombosis in those who are taking the combined pill

227

a. **True**   – For example, alcoholism is common in countries with cheap and readily available alcohol
b. **True**
c. **True**
d. **True**
e. **True**   – Though debated and difficult. If interested, see *Lancet* (1996) 347 : 31

228

a. **True**   – Needle marks, dilated pupils, goose flesh, vomiting, sneezing, running nose
b. **True**
c. **False** – Only authorized doctors can prescribe diamorphine for addiction
d. **True**   – Methadone, an opioid, will relieve symptoms
e. **False** – 40 mg or less/day is usually adequate. For a review of methadone maintenance, see *British Medical Journal* (1994) 309: 1997

229

a. **True**
b. **False**
c. **True**
d. **False**
e. **True**

230

Facts about alcohol:

a. The Department of Health recommends that the safe level of alcohol consumption is 3 units/day for a man and 2 units/day for a woman
b. A unit of alcohol is a glass of wine, a measure of spirits or a pint of beer
c. Given the same dose of alcohol, women have a higher level of alcohol in their blood
d. Chronic alcohol abuse can damage the heart
e. Excessive alcohol consumption in pregnancy can cause fetal abnormalities

230

a. **False** — This has been increased to 4 units for men and 3 for women. It is debated whether this is wise
b. **False** — Correct for wine and spirits, but a unit is half a pint of beer
c. **True** — Due to differences in distribution and metabolism within the body
d. **True**
e. **True** — Alcohol can cause growth and mental retardation and a characteristic facies. Many experts advise abstinence or only one unit/day in pregnancy

The local application of drugs

Many drugs are applied locally – the more active preparations are usually on prescription, but a number can be bought 'over the counter' without prescription. In the eye, drugs are usually applied as drops or ointment. On the skin, they are applied as ointments or lotions. Drugs may also be given systemically.

In treating eye conditions, locally applied drugs may be used for those affecting the surface of the eye, but they may also penetrate to the deeper structures. Nursing responsibilities include teaching patients how to manage their own drugs and to help with administration as required.

Disorders of the skin are numerous and many are treated by the patient with preparations purchased without prescription from the chemist. Nurses will be involved in the topical application of drugs both in and out of hospital. It is important therefore, to remember that using a wrong preparation, or over-treating, may exacerbate a lesion, and there is the ever-present risk of inducing hypersensitivity to the application.

231

A 12-year-old child has bacterial conjunctivitis (pink eye) which is to be treated with eye drops. Which of the following can apply?

a. One drop is instilled under the upper eyelid with the child looking downwards
b. The eye drops should be destroyed when the course is finished
c. Chloramphenicol 0.5% eye drops are commonly prescribed
d. This should be combined with 1% hydrocortisone eye drops
e. Eye drops should be instilled every 2 hours at the start of treatment

232

These drugs can damage the eye with prolonged use:

a. Ethambutol
b. Chloroquine
c. Isoniazid
d. Amiodarone
e. Corticosteroids

233

These drugs may worsen glaucoma in susceptible subjects:

a. Benzodiazepines
b. β Blockers
c. Tricyclic antidepressants
d. Atropine eye drops
e. Cimetidine

234

A patient comes to the A&E department with a small foreign body embedded in the cornea. To expedite removal, which is correct?

a. Cocaine eye drops (1%) are instilled in the eye
b. Oxybuprocaine eye drops (0.4%) are instilled in the eye
c. Cyclopentolate (0.5%) may be instilled to dilate the pupil
d. Fluorescein strips are applied to the eye to delineate the damage
e. Betnesol eye drops are given to minimize inflammation

231

a. **False** – They should be instilled in the lower fornix with the patient looking up
b. **True**
c. **True**
d. **False** – Corticosteroids can be dangerous unless supervised by an expert
e. **True**

232

a. **True** – Inflammation of the optic nerve
b. **True** – Retinal damage
c. **False**
d. **True** – Corneal deposits, but vision not affected
e. **True** – Cataracts, glaucoma

233

a. **False**
b. **False**
c. **True**
d. **True**
e. **False**

234

a. **False** – No longer used as it is too toxic
b. **True** – Local anaesthetic
c. **True** – Relieves spasm of ciliary muscle
d. **True**
e. **False** – It might increase the risk of infection

235

In the treatment of chronic open-angle glaucoma it is necessary to lower the intra-ocular pressure. This can be achieved by:

a. Timolol eye drops, which reduce fluid secretion
b. Sodium cromoglycate, which reduces inflammation
c. Pilocarpine eye drops, which constrict the pupil and increase the flow of intra-ocular fluid
d. Adrenaline eye drops, which decrease secretion and aid absorption
e. Tropicamide eye drops, which dilate the pupil

236

What advice would you give to a patient with very dry skin?

a. Emollients should be used regularly and include a bath oil as well as a moisturizing cream
b. Ointments are more effective than creams on very dry skin
c. Emollients should only be applied once daily
d. Aqueous cream can be used as a substitute for soap to clean the skin
e. Emollients should be rubbed vigorously into the skin

237

Local corticosteroids are widely used for various skin disorders and patients may seek your advice. Which of the following are true?

a. Hydrocortisone 1% cream is available without prescription
b. It should be applied four times daily
c. Betamethasone 0.1% is considerably more powerful than hydrocortisone 1%
d. No more than 2.0 g of betamethasone cream should be applied to each 9% of the body surface (e.g. face, neck and scalp) at any one time
e. Corticosteroid ointments are best applied to dry skin

235

a. **True** – But systemic absorption can occur, with cardiac effects
b. **False**
c. **True**
d. **True** – But dipivefrine may be better
e. **False** – If would make matters worse

236

a. **True**
b. **True**
c. **False** – Emollients should be applied as frequently as necessary to keep the skin hydrated
d. **True**
e. **False** – Creams and ointments should be smoothed onto the skin gently in the direction of hair growth. Vigorous rubbing can damage fragile, dry skin, with a risk of secondary infection and folliculitis occurring

237

a. **True**
b. **False** – No more than twice daily
c. **True**
d. **True**
e. **False** – It is more effective applied to hydrated skin

238

Prolonged and excessive application of corticosteroid preparations can cause:

a. Atrophy of the skin
b. Pigmentation of the skin
c. Local striae
d. Spread of local infection
e. Suppression of adrenal function

239

Which of the following skin reactions to a drug suggest that the disorder is serious and expert assistance must be obtained quickly?

a. Urticaria affecting the face and neck
b. Blistering of the lesions
c. Itching
d. High fever
e. Raised purpura

240

Sunscreens are now recommended to avoid sunburn and its attendant risks. In which situations are patients particularly liable to be photosensitive?

a. Those with vitamin D deficiency
b. Those being treated with β blockers
c. Those being treated with chlorpromazine
d. Those with systemic lupus erythematosus
e. Those being treated with amiodarone

238

a. **True**
b. **False**
c. **True**
d. **True**
e. **True** – Only with powerful steroids applied over wide areas

239

a. **True** – There is a risk of the oedema causing respiratory obstruction
b. **True** – It can progress to large areas of skin detachment (as in Stevens–Johnson syndrome and epidermal necrolysis)
c. **False** – Not necessarily a dangerous symptom
d. **True**
e. **True** – Suggests a vasculitis with possible organ involvement

240

a. **False** – Sunlight causes vitamin D to be formed in the skin
b. **False**
c. **True**
d. **True**
e. **True**

241

Certain drugs carry a high risk of causing skin sensitivity if applied locally and should be avoided if possible:

a. Penicillin
b. Chlortetracycline
c. Sulphonamides
d. Antihistamines
e. Acyclovir

241

a. **True**
b. **False** – One of the antibiotics least likely to cause a local reaction
c. **True**
d. **True** – Should not be used for more than three days
e. **False**

Disinfectants and insecticides

These substances fall into two broad groups: those intended as environmental disinfectants and those safe for application to the skin and mucous membranes (antiseptics). Nurses use both categories of disinfectant during their everyday work. They need to know the limitations of disinfectants in general and the specific properties of individual disinfectants, especially the range of organisms each is able to destroy and whether or not the disinfectant will damage particular types of equipment.

Some knowledge of insecticides is necessary to every health professional. Those used to treat bedding, houses, etc. may be highly poisonous chemicals which produce side-effects unless used properly. Others are used medically to treat infestations and it is important to ensure that instructions are followed properly if they are to be maximally effective.

242

Nurses will be well aware of the importance of sterility. Which of the following statements are true?

a. Disinfection is the destruction of vegetative bacteria and their spores
b. Sterilization is the destruction of vegetative bacteria and their spores
c. Antiseptics destroy vegetative bacteria and their spores
d. Detergents destroy vegetative bacteria and their spores
e. A good disinfectant may not be a good cleaning agent

243

The following are safe to apply to the skin:

a. Chlorhexidine
b. Povidone iodine 10%
c. Glutaraldehyde
d. Hypochlorites
e. Phenols

244

Infestation is still with us! Headlice can be treated with:

a. Malathion
b. Pyrethroids
c. A 2 hour contact with an insecticide is adequate
d. The application should be changed every 3 years to prevent the development of resistance
e. Prophylactic treatment should be carried out on contacts

242

a. **False** – It does not necessarily destroy the spores
b. **True**
c. **False** – Antiseptics usually destroy a narrow range of bacteria, but not spores
d. **False**
e. **True**

243

a. **True**
b. **True**
c. **False**
d. **True** – A 0.3% solution can be used for wound cleaning
e. **False**

244

a. **True**
b. **True**
c. **False** – Twelve hours contact is necessary to kill the eggs
d. **True**
e. **False** – Only treat infected subjects

Poisoning and its treatment

Intentional self-poisoning is a major health problem in the UK and is known to be growing in particular age groups. Nurses employed in a range of settings (A&E, acute wards and occasionally, long-term care) have to help patients and their families cope with the effects of attempted suicide in which drugs have been used. Similarly, accidental poisoning is a common problem among children. Paediatric nurses, school nurses and health visitors play an important part in helping families overcome their feelings of distress and recrimination when a child has swallowed drugs, as well as educating parents and teachers about the safe handling and storage of drugs.

245

The absorption of poison from the gut can be reduced by:

a. Giving activated charcoal by mouth
b. Colonic lavage
c. Giving an emetic
d. Gastric lavage
e. Haemoperfusion

246

In poisoning, which of these are correct?

a. Tricyclic antidepressants cause dilated pupils and cardiac arrhythmias
b. Aspirin causes depressed respiration and nystagmus
c. Paraquat (weedkiller) causes lung failure
d. Carbon monoxide usually causes confusion, coma and cyanosis or pallor
e. Morphine causes hypotension and hypothermia

247

In paracetamol poisoning:

a. Twenty 500 mg tablets can be dangerous
b. The antidote is ineffective if given more than 4 hours after the drug has been taken
c. An antidote is *N*-acetyl cysteine
d. 'Distalgesic' tablets contain paracetamol
e. Estimation of blood levels of the drug is an important part of management

245

a. **True** – The charcoal binds to the drug and prevents absorption
b. **False**
c. **True** – But little used these days
d. **True** – But declining in popularity
e. **False** – This does not alter absorption

246

a. **True**
b. **False** – Increased respiration, vomiting, tinnitus
c. **True**
d. **True** – The classical red colour of the skin is rare
e. **False** – Pin-point pupils and depressed respiration

247

a. **True**
b. **False** – Can be used up to 15 hours
c. **True**
d. **True** – Combined with a weak opioid
e. **True** – The blood level and time after dosing indicate the
probable outcome and best treatment